Developmental and Behavioral Complexities in Children

Developmental and Behavioral Complexities in Children provides students and professionals with an understanding of childhood mental health and developmental diagnoses through a series of qualitative vignettes alongside descriptions of clinical diagnoses and an overview of historical changes in the field.

A multidisciplinary, collaborative team of authors offers expertise based on questions received throughout their careers. The authors aim to ease some of the confusion that exists when navigating mixed messages about "typical" development, while providing state of the art information about specific diagnoses and clinical strategies and interventions that can be beneficial for children who may or may not meet criteria for a specific diagnosis.

The book gives clinicians and students a framework to guide caregivers in learning to decipher complicated messages around childhood developmental and mental health diagnoses and prepares them to support children's developmental, social, behavioral, and emotional growth.

Jo-Ann Blaymore Bier, MD is a retired developmental-behavioral pediatrician and former special educator, who was a senior associate at Boston Children's Hospital with board certifications in developmental-behavioral pediatrics and neurodevelopmental disabilities.

Theresa A. Johnson, MS, OTR/L is a registered, licensed occupational therapist at Perkins School for the Blind. She has extensive experience working with children in hospital, developmental clinic, and school settings.

Ellen Mullane, LICSW is a licensed independent clinical social worker who has worked with children and families in the medical setting, developmental clinic, and in the community.

"I would recommend this book to anyone teaching a course on child development. This book is essential for healthcare professionals who must understand diagnoses as well as the behaviors of children and factors that may be affecting development. The authors embrace family-centered care and interprofessional practice and present clinically relevant information in a clear way to support students' and early professionals' clinical reasoning."

Jane O'Brien, OTR, FAOTA, occupational therapist, University of New England, professor, retired

"A no-nonsense approach for teachers and other professionals in helping kids learn. Answering questions and providing suggestions to address a number of common issues that parents and teachers deal with on a daily basis."

Ralph Tripp, special education teacher and special education administrator, retired

"For the past decade, there has been an increased awareness of the vulnerability of children to stressors and behavioral challenges as well as the recognition of the diversity of learning and complex neurodevelopmental processes underlying learning at school. Bier and colleagues have written a much needed and important roadmap for health professionals, families, and children themselves. The interdisciplinary authors bring together updated scientific perspectives, best diagnostic practices, and practical management advice with a wealth of data driven and lifecourse experiences. In these times of difficulty accessing comprehensive coordinated care, they provide in a single book the sorely needed perspectives so that health professionals, parents, and children have a resource for their journeys toward independence."

Michael E. Msall, MD, professor of pediatrics University of Chicago Medicine and director of Developmental and Behavioral Pediatrics Fellowship Training Program

Developmental and Behavioral Complexities in Children

A Guide for Students and Clinicians

Jo-Ann Blaymore Bier,
Theresa A. Johnson, and
Ellen Mullane

Routledge
Taylor & Francis Group

NEW YORK AND LONDON

Designed cover image: Getty Images

First published 2026
by Routledge
605 Third Avenue, New York, NY 10158

and by Routledge
4 Park Square, Milton Park, Abingdon, Oxon, OX14 4RN

Routledge is an imprint of the Taylor & Francis Group, an informa business

ISBN: 9781041071549 (hbk)
ISBN: 9781041071563 (pbk)
ISBN: 9781003639121 (ebk)

DOI: 10.4324/9781003639121

Typeset in Bembo
by KnowledgeWorks Global Ltd.

Dedicated to the thousands of children and families who
allowed us the privilege of sharing their personal journeys.
You taught us everything we know and were the true inspiration
for this book.

Contents

Acknowledgements

After deciding to create a book based on our "life's work," it quickly became clear that synthesizing our knowledge and experiences into a book was going to be more challenging than we expected. Thank you to our colleagues who stepped up throughout this journey to assist us in attempting to put what was in our "heads" onto paper – Fred Dalzell, Libby Gormley, Lynn Plant, Kathy Siranosium, Dr. Elizabeth Wheeler, and Dr. Ann Zartler. A special thank you to Dr. Jane Clifford O'Brien, for sharing her extensive publication experience with us, and to Ralph Tripp, who generously shared his lifetime of educational expertise and compassionate knowledge of childhood behavior. And an especially huge thank you to Rebecca Bier, who stuck by our side throughout this process, always willing to lend support, academic knowledge, and fantastic writing skills to our work. We also truly appreciate the support of the rest of our family members – Rachel, Ben, Liya, Isaac, and Jon Bier (life partner and best friend), and Jeff and Violet Friedman, for their encouragement and willingness to review material and provide input and advice when requested; and Dennis Orsi and Meredith and Fiona Johnson for their support throughout this process. Finally, we are indebted to Routledge publishing, particularly our editors, Amanda Savage, who quickly supported the vision of this book, and Sophie Dracott, who closely guided us through this experience and provided timely and organized information and assistance throughout the publication process.

About the Authors

Jo-Ann Blaymore Bier, MD, MS is a recently retired developmental-behavioral pediatrician. She was a senior associate in Pediatrics at Boston Children's Hospital, with over 30 years of experience practicing developmental-behavioral pediatrics. Her board certifications included developmental-behavioral pediatrics and neurodevelopmental disabilities. Dr. Bier also earned a Master of Science degree in Special Education, with teaching certifications in secondary education and special education. She was an assistant professor of Pediatrics at Harvard Medical School, and continues to be a fellow of the American Academy of Pediatrics, a member of the Section of Developmental and Behavioral Pediatrics, and an elected member of the Society for Pediatric Research. Dr. Bier's primary areas of research included the developmental and psycho-social outcomes of high-risk infants and children with myelodysplasia. Dr. Bier has authored multiple publications in peer review journals and book chapters. She has been actively involved with the community in South Coast Massachusetts. She is currently on the board of directors of the Boys and Girls Club of Greater New Bedford, where she is also the director of their Health and Nutrition program.

Theresa A. Johnson, OT, MSOT, OTR is a supervising clinician and occupational therapist at Perkins School for the Blind with over 25 years of experience working with infants, children, and adults in a variety of settings including acute care hospitals, outpatient pediatric and child development clinics, public schools, and specialized schools for children with multiple disabilities. She earned a Master of Science degree in Occupational Therapy after completing a Bachelor of Science degree in Biology with a minor in Psychology. She has completed extensive continuing education coursework on childhood issues including topics such as positive discipline, crisis prevention, pediatric assessments, sensory processing, childhood disorders, and learning challenges. Her research interests have included the developmental outcomes of high-risk infants.

Ellen Mullane, LICSW, CCM is a graduate of Boston College Graduate School of Social Work. She has worked as a medical social worker for 40 years at Southcoast Health, Southcoast Children's Developmental Clinic, and in the community at Southcoast Visiting Nurse Association. She provides psychosocial assessments, intervention, short-term counseling, and collaboration of services with community agencies for children, adults, families, and care providers. She has been responsible for the development and presentation of lectures on topics related to child development, child welfare, domestic violence, substance abuse, and AIDS education.

Introduction

Contributing authors for this book include an occupational therapist, a social worker, and a developmental-behavioral pediatrician/former special education teacher. Our team worked for over 30 years with children and families in Southeastern Massachusetts. During that time, we helped thousands of families address concerns about their children's behavior and development and created plans to help children with a range of developmental abilities to grow, learn, and thrive. Although each child and family were unique, we often found ourselves responding to similar concerns –so much so that we started saying to one another, "We have to put this in a book!" Well, we did, and we hope that our many years of experience will help you expand your knowledge of child development and better prepare you to assist caregivers on their parenting journey.

As clinicians, we try to provide parents with what they need to help their children be successful and happy. But understanding children's behavior and development is not simple – the amazing journey of child development can be associated with questions, uncertainties, concerns, and sometimes, even doubts. Is this child okay? Are they learning at the rate they should be? Do they have the right skills for their age? Is this child acting too wild, too quiet, too distracted, too picky, too sensitive, too withdrawn, too rigid, etc., etc.? Throughout this book, you will find several examples of children who demonstrate skills or behaviors that may be a cause for concern. Although the examples in this book are fictional, they are based on stories the authors have heard multiple times. For example, let us talk about "Liam." Liam is three years old. He has always been very active. He loves running and jumping. His aunt noticed some behaviors that she felt may be concerning: Liam never seems to stay still long enough to look people in the eye or listen to what they are saying. He has always loved cars and trucks. He likes to line up his toy vehicles, which is one of the only times she sees him stay still. He can get agitated and even have a complete "melt down" if someone interferes with his play. Liam's aunt brought up her concerns with Liam's parents – is this a sign of autism? Is Liam just really into cars? Is Liam actually a gifted child with laser-like focus? Does he have ADHD? Liam's mom does not know how to answer these questions. She does some of her own research but finds an overwhelming amount of information that is difficult to decipher. She wants to better understand what signs she should look for, so she comes to you for advice.

Being a parent or caregiver can be stressful and can often result in seeking advice and guidance from professionals. As an advanced student or professional who may be early in your career, you will quickly realize that identifying what is typical in a child's development is not a task most parents feel well-equipped to handle. Parents, like Liam's mom, may do a great deal of research in child development and still not have a clear sense of what is typical development at certain ages and often hear conflicting advice. In addition, parents may be informed that "each child is different" and that "it is unfair to compare children" (particularly siblings), to one another. Therefore, when a parent observes differences in their child compared to their same aged peers or is informed by others that their child appears "different," this can result in apprehension about their child and/or their parenting skills. Parents may seek your professional opinion, as they attempt to better understand their unique child and navigate the overwhelming amount of available information.

As you prepare for, or advance, your professional career, you may also find that being able to reassure parents that their child's differences are within the range of typical development vs. a cause for concern, is not always that straightforward. You may be informed by parents that they have received confusing and sometimes conflicting information. You will try to avoid "missing" a diagnosis and also avoid "over diagnosing." Delaying a diagnosis can delay treatment and supportive services, but incorrectly labeling a child with a mental health diagnosis can also have negative consequences – for example, caregivers excusing inappropriate behaviors as a part of the child's diagnosis; treating the child as if he is different and facilitating the child's differences; and/or insisting that a child receive specific therapies that may not be needed.

This book will assist you in sorting out the possible significance of the behaviors and skills that caregivers may attribute to their children and describe to you. Differences in a child's behavior may be considered age-appropriate and not reflective of a specific diagnosis, even though intervention may be beneficial. In other instances, the differences may be suggestive of a specific developmental diagnosis. This book will explain why the field of child development is often not a "black and white" science. The way that children appear varies under different conditions and settings. Professionals may have varying thresholds for recommending intervention. Further, the criteria for developmental diagnoses sometimes change over time. Finally, this book provides information about supports and interventions that may be helpful in addressing children's challenges, whether or not they meet criteria for a specific diagnosis.

Inspired by over three decades working with parents and caregivers who asked questions, just like those from Liam's mom, the authors document a range of developmental behaviors considered "typical" and those that are likely symptoms of specific diagnoses. The book draws on perspectives in developmental pediatrics, social work, occupational therapy, and special education to unpack the black box of developmental-behavioral disorders. This book will provide practical and useful information for clinicians and advanced degree students who may be having difficulty sorting out the myriad developmental diagnoses that exist and looking for ways to help children's developmental, social, behavioral, and emotional growth. This book is not a "how-to" diagnose guide, but rather a resource for professionals who care for children and want to better understand the range of behaviors in children and aid in their development. It acknowledges different parenting styles and provides resources to help children with a range of developmental abilities to grow, learn, and thrive. This book aims to ease some of the confusion that can exist when navigating mixed messages about "typical" development, while providing state of the art information about specific diagnoses and providing clinical strategies and interventions that can be beneficial for children who may or may not meet criteria for a specific diagnosis.

CHAPTER 1

A Time Lapse View of Typical Child Development

It is not uncommon for a parent to express concerns or ask questions regarding their child's development. For some parents, concerns start during pregnancy or immediately following labor or delivery. A mother might wonder if her complicated pregnancy could impact her child's later development. A dad might have questions about the effect of his child's two-month stay in the special care nursery. Parents may express concerns about whether their own history of medical or mental health challenges will affect their child's future development and well-being. In addition, a parent who chooses to adopt a child may be apprehensive regarding the impact that the child's previous environment and genetic background may have on the child's future development. In order to respond to a caregiver's concerns about their child's development, it is useful to have a basic understanding of typical developmental trajectories. The goal of this first chapter is to provide a general overview of age ranges for typical development of childhood skills. It is designed to help you achieve a better understanding of child development during the early years, not just to list skills by age, but to provide information about how children are developing and gaining skills during each stage. The chapter also includes a description of infant reflexes and some developmental variations that can be observed in infants who were born prematurely.

Development Milestones are skills and behaviors that most typically developing children are able to exhibit within a specific age range. There are multiple lists and charts available describing the average ages children are expected to achieve various milestones. In 2022, the American Academy of Pediatrics (AAP) published the results of a working group who together revised its previous developmental surveillance checklist for primary care providers. The information was evidence-based and included skills that were relatively easy to observe and typically achieved by 75%

DOI: 10.4324/9781003639121-1

of children at specific age ranges in four developmental areas: cognitive, social-emotional, motor, and language/communication (Zubler et al., 2022).

The following developmental information includes data provided by the AAP working group, but it is presented in relatively broad age ranges and merges the various developmental areas. Our goal is to present a "time-lapsed moving picture" of typical childhood developmental trajectories. In addition, we attempt to incorporate the concept that differentiating a normal developmental trajectory from causes for developmental concern can sometimes be less related to **what** a child is able to do at a certain age than to **the way** they are performing some of those skills. Finally, it should be noted that some children who do not appear to be meeting milestones within a specific age range may not ultimately be diagnosed with a developmental disorder; conversely, although achieving milestones "on time" is reassuring, it may not definitively rule out a future disorder.

EARLY INFANCY (0 TO 3 MONTHS)

A typical newborn baby enters this world with many important capabilities already developed. Many of their skills are considered "reflexes." A reflex is a movement that is "automatic" or involuntary. For example, a newborn will automatically suck if a finger or nipple is placed into their mouth. From an evolutionary perspective, newborn reflexes are considered "survival reflexes," as their existence helps a newborn locate and ingest nutrition and maintain physical contact with their caretaker. Some newborn reflexes disappear in weeks, some after a few months, and some transition into voluntary behaviors. Newborn reflexes include the following.

- Rooting: If a newborn's cheek or mouth is stroked, they will automatically turn their head, enabling them to find the nipple for feeding. The infant will turn their head from side to side until they position the nipple in their mouth to suck.
- Sucking: When a nipple (or other object, such as a finger) is placed in an infant's mouth, they will automatically begin to suck. Sucking is even observed prior to birth – for example, an ultrasound may show a fetus sucking on their thumb. An infant's sucking pattern becomes more proficient, rhythmical, and eventually voluntary over time.
- Moro: If a young infant's head shifts positions or falls backwards fairly suddenly, or the infant is startled, the infant will extend their arms, legs, and neck and then bring their arms quickly together. This reflex typically disappears by about two months of age.

- Palmar grasp: Newborn infants will reflexively "grasp" something placed into or stroking the palm of their hand – for example, an adult's finger.
- Stepping: When held vertically so that the soles of the feet have contact with a surface, the infant makes a "walking"-like movement with their legs. This reflex typically lasts only a couple of months
- Tonic neck reflex, also referred to as the Asymmetric tonic neck reflex: This is sometimes described as the "fencing" reflex. When an infant's head is turned to one side, the arm on that side will straighten, and the opposite arm will bend at the elbow. This reflex may not be observed strongly and/or consistently and disappears at about 5 to 7 months of age.

Newborn infants are able to turn their heads from side to side when they are placed prone/on their abdomen. This is an important skill that allows the infant to keep their nose and mouth clear from a surface for breathing. It is the recommendation of the American Academy of Pediatrics to place all infants on their back for sleeping (Moon et al., 2022), however having the opportunity to spend time on their stomachs during wakeful hours of the day throughout the first three months of life is very important. Time spent prone, often referred to as "tummy time", is critical for infants. Tummy time allows infants to build neck strength and range of motion, which results in the advancement of head control skills and the baby's ability to support their own head in various positions. Tummy time also helps build the foundation for other motor skill development by stretching and strengthening the muscles of the arms, abdomen, and back, which will lead to the skills of rolling over, crawling, and getting into a hands and knees position in later months. The early development of hand skills is also seen toward the latter part of this three-month time period and into the next period beginning at four months, including infants bringing their hands to the middle of their bodies and to their mouths.

Young infants use their eyes and ears to begin to learn about their world. During this stage of infancy, babies typically are interested in looking at faces and begin to smile at people. They also begin using their eyes to follow people or objects. They are often alerted by sounds in the environment (hearing testing is recommended before a newborn infant is discharged from the hospital). Infants from 0 to 3 months enjoy being spoken to and sung to as they are advancing their seeing, hearing, and thinking skills. They may also begin to make cooing sounds as they are learning to use their voices. Providing a rich environment that includes many social interactions with caregivers allows the infant many opportunities to practice and enhance these early social and cognitive skills.

MIDDLE INFANCY (4 TO 9 MONTHS)

Infants at this stage are now able to use some of the skills established in the earlier months to interact with the people and objects in their environment. Cooing vowel sounds at four months of age become more extensive. The start of some consonant and consonant-vowel sounds can be observed as an infant progresses through middle infancy. During this time period, infants often use their babbling playfully when interacting with caregivers, enjoy looking at themselves in a mirror, blow "raspberries" by sticking out their tongue and blowing, and laugh interactively.

The improved visual skills of 4- to 9-month-old infants allow them to recognize familiar people and even begin to mimic facial movements and expressions in social interactions. They can visually follow caregiver's movements, as well as the movement of objects/toys in their environment. By nine months, infants often begin to enjoy social games, particularly games with a predictable, repetitive component such as "peek-a-boo" (the beginning of the development of object permanence – "out of sight, NOT out of mind"); they respond by looking when their name is called, react when a caregiver leaves, and can become more shy and sometimes fearful around strangers.

Infants begin to demonstrate more coordinated and smoother arm and hand movements and can pair eye and hand movement together to reach for and grasp objects. They can bring their hands and toys to their mouths, hold and shake objects, and are even beginning to manipulate objects by rotating them and passing them to the opposite hand. By nine months, infants will typically look for an object, such as a spoon, when it has dropped to the floor.

Movement skills emerge at this stage. Infants are able to lift their heads, arms, and legs off of a surface when they are prone. They can typically roll from their backs to their stomachs and vice versa. They may begin using their arms and legs to scoot themselves forward in an "army-crawl" manner during the latter-half of this stage and may even get onto their hands and knees and begin rocking. As infants progress through this stage, moving their bodies becomes a routine part of their play. They often experiment with moving simply for the sake of moving (for example, rolling over and over) or as a means to get something in their environment such as a toy or a caregiver. Most infants begin moving by creeping on their hands and knees during the latter part of this stage. When supported in a standing position on a firm surface, the infants will push down through their legs bearing weight on their feet. Sitting skills are also emerging at this stage – infants can often sit with the support of their hands on the surface in front of their bodies, and later without the need for support.

During this stage infants benefit from having a safe space to play, explore, and move such as a playpen or gated, padded play area during the day. Having many opportunities to practice their movement skills, strengthen their body and limb muscles, and explore simple, safe objects with their hands and mouths allows the infant to develop age-appropriate foundation skills. Frequent social interactions with caregivers remain very important at this stage as the infant is learning to read and respond to facial expressions and voices. Social interactions allow the infant to build communication skills, emotional connections, and even motor skills.

LATE INFANCY THROUGH TODDLERHOOD (10 TO 18 MONTHS)

The foundational skills that were developed during the first six to nine months of life are the building blocks used to allow vast changes to occur during the 10- to 18-month period. Infants go from being completely dependent on caregivers to meet all of their needs and desires, to being able to communicate their needs and desires in a variety of ways and to physically act on their environment to achieve some of those needs and desires themselves during this stage.

In the 10- to 18-month stage, infants become much more skilled at identifying familiar people. They are often afraid of strangers and may have difficulty separating from their caregiver. They become much more interactive with caregivers as noted by their ability to imitate gestures or words, to take turns in simple songs or games, to make a request with a word or gesture (for example, put their arms up in the air when wanting to be held), and/or to follow simple directions with gestures provided (for example, "wave bye-bye" or "give a kiss"). They often enjoy repeating familiar games over and over again, such as "pat-a-cake." They are developing more ways to interact with caregivers such as pointing to objects of interest and/or showing objects they have, and following directions (for example, "give me that"). Infants also use their voices more readily during this stage as another way to interact with caregivers. Babbling becomes extensive and evolves into familiar words (for example, "mama," "dada," "baby," "ball," a sibling's name) and word approximations (for example, "baba" for "bottle"; "nana" for "banana"), with a gradual increase in the number of words, and finally two-word phrases (for example, "My toy!"; "What's that?")

Hand-use skills and movement skills also greatly advance during this stage. Infants typically become independent in getting in and out of a sitting position, and learn to get around on their hands and knees. They learn to use a stable object to pull themselves into a standing position, and then begin using a side-stepping motion to walk while holding furniture or the side of a playpen or play-yard (also referred to as "cruising"). As their movement and strength improve, they are able to balance while standing, and eventually learn to move from one place to another by taking forward steps without support. Infants at this stage are able to pick large things up with two hands together. Their ability to pick up small things between their thumb and index finger becomes more precise. They are able to use both hands together to pull loose-fitting items apart, and to put items into a container and take them out. Filling objects into containers and then dumping the objects out, and then repeating this task often becomes an enjoyable activity. Young toddlers continue to refine their cognitive and motor skills, eventually developing the ability to stack cubes and other objects.

Let Us Re-visit Reflexes – Specifically, Postural Reflexes

As an infant develops, new reflexes appear that protect them as they acquire more advanced skills. **Postural reflexes**, also sometimes referred to as "protective reflexes", help infants maintain their equilibrium and posture, assisting them in staying upright when their body is thrown off balance. While newborn reflexes are initiated in the brainstem, most of the postural reflexes arise from more advanced/mature areas of the central nervous system. Postural reflexes can remain as they integrate into a child's movement patterns – for example, an individual's hand will automatically go forward in response to tripping and falling. Both "righting" and "equilibrium" reflexes/responses are considered postural reflexes, as they assist infants in maintaining correct alignment and posture, keeping their body aligned with their center of gravity, and maintaining balance both during movement and also while still.

- Neck and head righting reflexes: Although many of the postural reflexes develop during the second half of an infant's first year; the head and neck righting reflexes develop earlier. These reflexes enable an infant to keep their head in midline. Neck righting results in rotation of the body in response to head rotation, and head righting enables an infant to hold their head up when prone and keep their head in line with their body when they are pulled up from supine (on their back) to a sitting position.

- Body righting reflex: This reflex modifies the neck righting reflex, as the body will "right" itself, keeping the body well positioned, independent of the head's position.
- Segmental rolling reflex: As an infant matures, they transition from neck righting to body righting to segmental rolling, during which the body rolls in "segments" rather than in a single "block."
- Landau reflex: When an infant is held under the abdomen horizontal to the floor, their head, legs, and spine will extend like an "airplane." The reflex is observed from about three months until about a year.
- Propping reactions: If a seated infant is tilted to one side, their arm will extend to prevent them from falling over.
- Parachute reflex: This reflex presents at about eight months. If an infant is held and moved toward the floor, their arms will straighten, as if to protect them from falling.

Of note, the protective reflex when an infant is tilted off their center of gravity towards the back, is typically observed later than those to the front and sides.

MIDDLE TODDLERHOOD (19 TO 24 MONTHS)

Children who are 19 to 24 months of age have a strong foundation of knowledge about things in their environment. They know who familiar people are (for example, family members, family friends, etc.), what many familiar objects are (for example, phone, toothbrush, keys, etc.), and how to interact with many things in their environment (for example, throw a ball, sit on a stool, hand a cup to an adult, etc.). An increased awareness of themselves and their own bodies is emerging at this stage. They can typically point to basic body parts on themselves. They may also show interest in others by watching them and wanting what they have. A 20-month-old child playing in a sandbox may see another child scoop with a shovel, then go over to that child and take the shovel from his or her hand. Such behavior is typical because a child at this stage has an awareness of others and the knowledge of how to use the desired object, but may not yet have developed the social skills to wait for the shovel to become available or to request a turn.

At this stage children can use verbal language and gestures to communicate and engage with others. They can imitate an action they observe others doing (for example, bring a spoon to a doll's mouth). They can also follow simple directions such as "Sit down here please" or "Get the ball and put it in the basket." Children at this stage of development generally have many words that they use regularly. They begin labeling common objects in books or in their environment, often pointing at and naming things simultaneously. It is typical for children to begin putting two words together to make a simple phrase (for example, "baby eat," "go park," etc.). Temper tantrums may emerge at this stage as well. Communication skills are developing but can be limited; frustration related to communication limitations and/or physical limitations can lead to temper tantrums. Understanding a young toddler's challenges and frustrations can make it easier for caregivers to deal with, and resolve, these types of tantrums.

As children at this stage have developed more awareness of themselves and others and have more advanced cognitive and motor skills, they begin to explore their environment on their own. However, they usually will not stray too far from their familiar caregiver, checking in often either by physically touching the caregiver or visually looking at the caregiver for reassurance. Fear or uneasiness with strangers may also be present, particularly in new situations or environments. Children at this stage typically seek to share their interest in something with a caregiver. They often hold an object out toward a caregiver. When holding an item up in this way, the child wants to share her experience with the caregiver, but is usually not looking for the caregiver to take the item. Rather, the child would like the caregiver to comment and acknowledge her interest in what she is holding. The child will likely smile, laugh, and/or continue playing if the caregiver comments by saying, for example, "That is a nice truck!" or "You made a big tower!" Children frequently seek feedback from caregivers in this way and are eager to have a caregiver acknowledge their success or pleasure. The emergence of simple pretend play is also seen at this stage. Children begin to feed a doll, as they have seen others do, or "drink" from a toy cup.

During this stage children are independent walkers and begin to enjoy developing their movement skills further for activities such as climbing on/off low furniture or steps, pulling toys while walking, and even running. Balance continues to advance as children physically move on and around objects in their environment. At this stage, children often enjoy playing with push toys, child-sized shopping carts or doll strollers, and being pushed on simple ride-on toys. Improvements in their large motor skills lead to an increase in independence with daily activities such as getting a desired toy off a low shelf, helping caregivers with dressing by moving their arms and legs into and out of clothing, and feeding themselves with utensils. Smaller, fine motor skills continue to improve as well. Children often begin making dots with a crayon, then scribbling with crayons, putting smaller items into a container, and holding utensils to feed themselves.

LATE TODDLERHOOD (2 TO 3 YEARS)

The "terrible twos," as they are notoriously called, are actually an exciting period of environmental exploration and desired independence. Two-year-olds are eager to imitate actions they have seen others do. If they see their caregiver is cooking, they want to use pots and pans too. They will often reach into someone else's personal space to take the toy or object that person is using in order to use it themselves. Two-year-olds are often excited to see other children, but will often play near them (known as parallel play) rather than playing with them. The skill of playing with peers develops toward the later part of this stage and usually begins with simple games such as chase or imitative games (for example, jumping and stomping together). Two-year-olds are able to understand familiar words more readily, including names of familiar people, body parts, and everyday objects. They are also able to use more words to express themselves, speaking in phrases and simple sentences.

Two-year-olds are steady on their feet and are capable of running, getting increasingly faster as they head toward age three. Other motor skills that emerge during this year include the ability to jump with two feet and to kick a ball. At this age, children can walk up and down stairs while holding onto a railing or an adult's hand; they may begin going up and down without holding, but will likely place both feet on each step. Climbing becomes a common activity for two-year-olds. They are able to climb on and off most furniture independently and can typically climb the steps of a small slide with supervision. Additional skills acquired in the second year include throwing a ball overhand, stacking several small blocks, holding utensils and crayons, and helping in self-care activities such as brushing their teeth. They often begin using one hand more than the other, although the full development of a dominant hand can take several years for some children.

PRESCHOOL (3 TO 5 YEARS)

The preschool years are a period of exciting discovery, independence, and also social interaction with peers. For children in this age group, their world is expanding, and most preschoolers are eager to use the skills they have developed to become a part of this new, larger world. During this stage of development, children are shifting from being self-centered to having a greater awareness of others around them.

At this stage, children become more interested in playing with other children than playing alone. Their play shifts from being parallel to other children (playing near them) to being integrative (interacting with other children during play). Their play also becomes more creative with lots of role playing and make-believe concepts – for example, saying things like, "You be the baby and I'll be the mommy" within pretend play. Preschoolers love trying out other roles and imitating jobs (for example, playing doctor, school, post-office, etc.). Children at this age have developed language skills and fundamental knowledge that allow them to interact with other children and adults beyond their families. They are beginning to cooperate with other children and develop social interactive skills such as turn taking and simple negotiation.

Pre-academic skills seen in children at this stage of development include counting, knowledge of colors, sorting objects by categories, and identification of numbers and letters. Children at this age are also able to draw "primitive" pictures. Preschoolers can typically state their first and last name, and can recall simple familiar songs and/or stories.

Children at this stage of development enjoy using their newly developed motor skills to do things independently. They are able to use crayons, deftly use spoons and forks, cut with scissors, and even pour a small drink (although this one might be a little messy at times). The emergence of a dominant hand typically becomes clear at this stage. Greater independence is seen in self-care skills such as dressing/undressing, tooth-brushing, and toileting skills. Skillful large motor actions can also be seen such as hopping on one foot, riding a tricycle, and catching a bounced ball.

ELEMENTARY SCHOOL (6 TO 11 YEARS)

During the elementary school age range, growth and development continue as children refine and enhance cognitive skills, motor skills, communication, and social-emotional skills. Academically, children in the early years of elementary school are working on learning basic skills such as math facts and reading. During the later elementary years, children are utilizing those basic skills within their learning. They are able to apply the fundamental principles they learned previously to more advanced material in order to gain more knowledge. In terms of social-emotional development, there is a transition that happens from being very family-focused to being more friend/school community focused. Elementary school children begin building independence from their parents/families. Friendships become more complex and more important in helping children determine their place in the wider world beyond their home life. Additionally, significant physical changes occur as children grow and move toward puberty. They likely become more aware of their bodies and begin thinking about the future rather than just the here and now. Physical skills (fine motor and gross motor) are generally mature and well established at this age. This developmental maturity allows children to hone in on advancing specific motor skills around their areas of interest such as sports, arts, playing an instrument, etc.

A WORD ABOUT MIDDLE- AND HIGH SCHOOL-AGED CHILDREN (11 TO 18 YEARS)

The main focus of this book is the development of young children from birth through elementary school – this time period is chock full of milestones, growth, and the advancement of many, many skills. Of course, there is also enormous growth and development as children continue to develop through middle school and beyond, strengthening and sharpening the foundational skills they built during their early years. Middle school and high school years represent a time of tremendous change. Major cognitive development, including critical thinking, reasoning, and self-reflection, occurs during this time. These pre-teen and teenage years also reveal in-depth social-emotional advances as children develop their own identity and determine their place in the world, not only within their family, but also within their peer group and their community at large. Because of the complexity and magnitude of the physical, cognitive, and emotional advancements during this time period, it was decided to limit the major focus of this book to the development and behavior of children through pre-adolescence.

CHILDREN BORN PREMATURELY

The length of a full-term pregnancy is considered to be about 40 weeks long. Children born at 37, 38, or 39 weeks gestation are also considered "full-term," but infants born before that time are considered premature. When an infant is born early, the expectations for their development are typically "corrected" for their prematurity; that is, the infant's development and skills reflect the age they would be if they had been born full term. For example, a child who was born at 31 weeks gestation was born nine weeks (about two months) prematurely. The child's skills four months after her birth would be expected to be more similar to a two-month-old infant instead of a four-month-old infant. In addition, the quality of the infant's skills may differ from a child who was born at term. Instead of being in their mother's womb during the latter part of the pregnancy, these infants were in the hospital, which can affect their patterns of development. For example, since premature infants spend more time lying on their backs vs. floating in their mother's womb during the latter part of the 40 weeks, they sometimes develop a tendency to extend their shoulders backwards. All the interventions recommended for infants who were born full term are therefore even more important for infants who were born early, including "tummy time," supporting their head to keep it midline when in a sitting position, and encouraging them to reach out with both hands.

Children who were born prematurely are considered to be at a higher risk for developmental and behavioral challenges. Both the earlier a child is born and the more complications the child experienced after birth increase this risk. Based on their history, children who were born premature may be referred to early intervention and may be enrolled in a neonatal follow-up program to monitor their developmental progress.

AUTHORS' COMMENTARY

Observing a child as they develop and guiding them on their journey of growth and development can sometimes be challenging but can also be extraordinarily exciting and rewarding. It is not uncommon for caregivers to express concerns that their child is not reaching developmental milestones at the accepted times, or they may have specific concerns about the child's unusual, quirky, or challenging behaviors. Sometimes sorting out whether a child is taking a slightly different developmental path or may actually be presenting with a specific diagnosis can be complex. Several chapters in this book will provide you with information that can assist you in sorting out these concerns.

BIBLIOGRAPHY

Altmann, T. R., & Hill, D. L. (Eds) (2019). *Caring for Your Baby and Young Child: Birth to Age 5 – 7ᵗʰ edition*. Elk Grove Village, IL: American Academy of Pediatrics.

American Academy of Pediatrics. Ages and Stages. https://www.healthychildren.org.

Brazelton T. B., & Sparrow J. D. (2009). *Touchpoints – Birth to Three*. New York City, NY: Hachette Book Group.

Brown D. F., & Knowles T. (2014). *What Every Middle School Teacher Should Know – 3ʳᵈ edition*. Portsmouth, NH: Heinemann Educational Books.

Moon R. Y., Carlin R. F., & Hand I. (2022). Sleep-related infant deaths: updated 2022. Recommendations for reducing infant deaths in the sleep environment. From the American Academy of Pediatrics Policy Statement. *Pediatrics*, 150(1): e2022057990. https://doi.org/10.1542/peds.2022-057990.

Schmitt B. (2024). Newborn Reflexes and Behavior. *Pediatric Patient Education*. American Academy of Pediatrics Publications. https://doi.org/10.1542/ppe_schmitt_178.

Zubler J. M., Wiggins L. D., Macias M. M., Whitaker T. M., Shaw J. S., Squires J. K., Pajek J. A., Wolf R. B., Slaughter K. S., Broughton A. S., Gerndt K. L., Mlodoch B. J., & Lipkin P. H. (2022). Evidence-informed milestones for developmental surveillance. *Pediatrics*, 140(3): e2021052138. https://doi.org/10.1542/peds.2021-052138.

CHAPTER 2

General Behavioral Strategies

Children's behavior can be thought of as a form of communication – they are trying to tell you "something" – is it that they are frustrated, angry, or sad? Trying to find the meaning behind a behavior or the "trigger" for a behavior can be helpful. "Listening" to what a child is trying to communicate can teach them mutual respect. However, it can sometimes be difficult to understand the meaning of, or trigger behind, difficult behaviors – sometimes the behaviors seem to "take on a life of their own." Coping with children's behavioral challenges can be overwhelming for everyone involved in the child's life (Tripp, 2021).

If a child has multiple problematic behaviors, it can be helpful to request that a caregiver make a list starting with the behavior that is the most disruptive, i.e., the problem that has the most negative impact on the child's and the rest of the family's functioning. It is typically not possible to work on improving all of the child's challenges at the same time. Prioritizing the greatest challenge will allow you to help the caregiver target and focus on a specific area. By breaking behavior into smaller components, this approach can make addressing the challenges more manageable. It can also build momentum in order to tackle other challenges as the caregivers successfully manage one at a time.

Finally, it is important to note that any regression in a child's behavior, development, eating, or sleeping patterns should be discussed with the child's primary care physician to explore possible medical etiologies - for example, infections, iron deficiency, lead ingestion, etc.

DOI: 10.4324/9781003639121-2

EXAMPLES OF SOME BEHAVIORAL STRATEGIES TO DISCUSS WITH CAREGIVERS

Modeling and Reinforcing Positive Behaviors

Adults should attempt to model appropriate responses to frustrating situations. If a child responds to situations in a positive manner, they should be celebrated and the behavior reinforced.

Structure and Consistency

All children benefit from structure and consistency in their daily routines. Some families are more structured than others, and it is not feasible for parents to be structured and consistent in their parenting 100% of the time. Keeping a visual schedule on a dry erase board or bulletin board, possibly including pictures, can be comforting to a child. Maintaining a consistent and structured bedtime routine built around relaxing rather than stimulating activities can help to decrease sleep difficulties.

Knowing what to expect typically lessens anxiety, but all children also need to learn strategies to cope with changes in their routine. Teaching these strategies before a large change occurs can be helpful. For example, try creating simple stories about a change in routine, such as a school vacation day, visiting a friend, or having dinner in a restaurant, and telling this story multiple times to a child to help him learn strategies to cope with changes and transitions.

Simplify the Environment When Possible, Including Decreasing Stimulation

Over-stimulation, including excessive noise or lights, visual clutter, etc., can increase anxiety and make some children feel overwhelmed. Whenever possible, remove unnecessary items, sounds, or lights to create a quieter, less stimulating environment.

Create a Place for Children to "Cool Off" During Tantrums – a Space That Is Safe, Where the Child Will Not Receive Attention

Setting aside a "cool off" or "time-out" space in the home that is only used when a child is having a tantrum or demonstrating inappropriate behavior can be helpful. The space should not be frightening, locked, over-stimulating, or potentially dangerous, nor should it be in the child's bedroom or toy room if possible. A designated area in a carpeted room such as the foyer can work well, or even something as simple as a soft chair in a quiet area. If a child is initially resistant to staying in the area, a parent should request (once) that they stay, or physically place the child back in the area stating (again, only once), "Time for you to relax in your cool-off space."

Speak Simply

For younger children or children with communication delays, speak in single words combined with a gesture. During mealtimes, for example, pointing to the milk while looking at your child and asking "milk?" may encourage them to respond.

Use "First/Then" Language Whenever Possible

Phrase instructions as, "First _____ (non-preferred activity/item), then _____ (preferred activity/item)." For example, you can help a child understand the expectation by saying, "First you put on your shoes, then we can go outside to play."

Redirect the Child Whenever Possible

If a child is demonstrating a behavior that is not acceptable or is atypical – for example, a self-stimulatory behavior – attempting to redirect the child's attention to another activity is appropriate. If a child is becoming frustrated, or you can tell that he may be building up to a tantrum, distracting him with a new activity may prevent the tantrum from occurring. It is often easier to stop a negative behavior before it escalates than it is to stop once it is happening.

Planned Ignoring

If redirection is unsuccessful, parents should make every effort to ignore inappropriate behaviors, particularly when escalation is occurring. Do not make eye contact or speak. Instead, walk away if safety allows. Try to stay neutral and calm, and do not attempt to negotiate.

Restating the Expectation

A parent can remind their child of how they want him to behave – for example, "I would be happy to help you with that toy when you are using a quiet voice and gentle hands."

Reinforce Appropriate Behavior

Verbally praise the child when he is following the schedule and the rules at home. Give praise that describes the desired behavior – for example, "I'm proud of the way you put all of your toys away before going outside."

Provide Opportunities for Movement

Many children will be better able to engage in a sit-down activity if they are provided with a movement activity first. Providing movement breaks during an activity may also improve the child's ability to complete the activity successfully.

Model Expected Behaviors

Use an appropriate tone of voice, be respectful, show empathy, and apologize when appropriate.

Consistency

Keep expectations the same as often as possible – for example, if the rule is no snacks before dinner, try to avoid giving in to requests for snacks at that time.

Natural Consequences

Use natural consequences to encourage desired behavior – for example, "If your basketball shirt stays on your floor instead of in the laundry basket, it will not get washed before your next game."

Humor and Playfulness

Use humor or playfulness to encourage your child to do what is needed – for example, "Who can put those blocks away the fastest?"

Find Productive Ways to Express Frustration

Help your child find safe, productive ways to express frustration or anger – for example, drawing, writing, kneading play dough, etc.

Support a Feeling of Being in Control

Give children control by building choices into the expectations – for example, "Do you want to do your math homework first or your spelling homework?"

Break Down Tasks

Break challenging tasks, such as cleaning their room, into smaller, more manageable pieces – for example, have them clean the desk area before dinner and the closet after dinner.

Offer Alternatives for Negative Behaviors

"You may not color on the walls, but here are some paper grocery bags you can spread out and color on."

Use Songs

Sing a familiar song or a made-up song to help engage your child in less desirable tasks.

Use Positive Language

When possible, state your directions in a positive rather than a negative way – for example, "Let's walk around the puddle," instead of, "Don't jump in the puddle."

Create an Environment that Limits the Temptation or Opportunity for Negative Behavior Whenever Possible

For example, put extra snack foods out of reach, have parental codes on TVs, etc.

Reduce Behavioral Triggers

Whenever possible provide snacks and/or sufficient sleep to limit things like hunger and fatigue which can make cooperation and compliance more difficult.

Help the Child Create a Solution to the Problem

Ask the child what can be done to fix a problem or to prevent it from happening in the future.

Give Yourself a Time-Out

Sometimes you may need to step back and take a few minutes to calm your own emotions before trying to correct a negative behavior.

HANDOUT FOR CAREGIVERS

Common Questions

I am unable to take my child into the mall or even the grocery store. If he sees something he wants, and I don't get it for him, he has a major tantrum/meltdown. What should I do?

A child can become upset when he is unable to have something that he requested. Some children have a decreased ability to cope with being told "no." Although most children can eventually understand that their tantrum will not be successful in obtaining what they want, it can still be very difficult handling a child having a tantrum in a public place. A systematic way to try to address this behavior is to explain to a child beforehand that something special will happen if they are well behaved in the specific environment, and then only stay for a very limited amount of time (possibly only five minutes). This allows the child a chance to be successful. Then praise your child for good behavior and provide the agreed upon reward (for example, a sticker, a special dessert, etc.). Gradually increasing the amount of time spent in the environment would be the next step, each time attempting to limit the visit enough to avoid a tantrum. For children with developmental challenges, including those that are nonverbal, you can start by walking in the store and walking out, praising the child and giving a sticker, each time increasing the time spent by a very short amount. While this technique might not allow you to get your grocery shopping done, it is giving your child the chance to practice and master the skill of going to the store without having a tantrum.

What should I do about a child who is very resistant to potty/toileting training?

A child's teacher and therapist/counselor can provide assistance in attempting to bowel- and bladder-train your child.

Some recommendations that may be beneficial:

- Begin by changing your child's pull-up or diaper in the bathroom, and praise your child for cooperating. Clap after you flush a bowel movement that has been placed in the toilet.
- Be aware of when your child typically has a bowel movement during the day.
- Have your child sit on the potty at regular intervals during the day.
- If your child urinates on the potty but will not have bowel movements on the potty, do not refuse to allow them to have bowel movements in a diaper or pull-up, as this can result in stool withholding.

- Try not to make potty-training a battle with your child (it is likely that your child will "win" the battle).
- Save one special song or story for potty time only.
- Use a sticker chart or other reward system for successes in the bathroom to help motivate your child.

What should I do about a child who resists going to sleep at night and often awakens and comes into my bed?

Create a structured, relaxing bedtime routine and do your best to implement the routine every night. Reading a book, playing soft music, and keeping the room fairly dark with possibly only a night-light are helpful components of a bedtime routine.

It is best not to have a television in your child's room, and electronic devices should be turned off at least an hour before bedtime.

Although this can often be challenging, teaching your child to fall asleep without a parent/guardian present should be a goal. When anyone wakes up in the middle of the night, they will have difficulty falling back to sleep if their pillow is not on their bed. Similarly, if a child falls asleep cradled in their parent's arms, or even just having a parent near their bed, and they wake up during the night, they will have difficulty putting themselves back to sleep without their parent present. Providing your child with a "transition object" such as a stuffed animal can be helpful, as the object will be there to soothe them back to sleep if they wake.

My child eats the same things over and over and is resistant to trying new foods. He only eats the same brand of his preferred foods. If I insist that he try a non-preferred food, he sometimes gags. How can I help him become less picky?

If your child is not gaining weight and his pediatrician is concerned about his weight gain or growth, an evaluation is indicated.

If your child's growth is not problematic, then working with a feeding therapist can be explored. In addition, the following strategies may be helpful.

- To introduce new foods or known non-preferred foods, use a very gradual presentation. Pay attention to your child's cues and progress at your child's pace.
- Praise your child for even allowing non-preferred foods on his plate; after this is comfortable, praise your child for imitating touching the non-preferred food to his lips, then tasting, etc.
- The more control and input your child has in the feeding strategy, the more likely it will be met with success – for example, ask, "Do you want spinach or peas?"

- Model dipping foods into various purees, and if your child imitates this activity, provide praise.
- Encourage your child to "assist" with food preparation – for example, helping to spoon foods into serving bowls will improve your child's comfort with the food.
- Allow your child to help plan a menu, which may increase the likelihood that your child will accept the foods that he included on the menu.
- Attempt to make mealtime fun – for example, request that your child help to use a cookie cutter to turn bread, cheese, deli meats into fun shapes and sizes. Build on pre-academic concepts: "Can you eat a bite of brown food now?" or "Eat the food that is the shape of a circle." Use fictional characters such as superheroes to encourage trials of new foods.
- Encourage healthy eating habits.

Final note: Strategies that are recommended for typical children are also useful, and can be even more important, for children with developmental and behavioral challenges.

BIBLIOGRAPHY

Ayres, A. J., & Robbins J. (1979). *Sensory Integration and the Child*. Los Angeles, Calif: Western Psychological Services.

Nelsen, J. (2013). *Positive Discipline*. New York City: Ballantine Books.

Phelan, T. W. (2020). *1-2-3 Magic:3-Step Discipline for Calm, Effective, and Happy Parenting: Effective discipline for Children 2–12*. San Francisco, CA: Blurb, Incorporated.

Toomey, K. A., & Sundseth, E. (2011). SOS approach to feeding. *Perspectives of Swallowing and Swallowing Disorders (Dysphagia)*, 20(3): 82–87. https://doi.org/10.1044/sasd20.3.82.

Tripp R. (2021). *Angry Kids are Telling Us Something. Presentation*. New Bedford, MA: Little People's College, New Bedford. MA.

CHAPTER 3

Intellectual Developmental Disorder or Just a Little Delayed?

To more fully understand many current developmental diagnoses, we feel that it is important to have an understanding of how terminology and societal views evolved in the field of child development and developmental disabilities. So, before we describe three children who present with developmental concerns, let us travel down some important and relevant historical paths.

Individuals with intellectual disabilities have been described throughout history, including by Hippocrates in the 5th century BCE. During the 17th century an English physician, Thomas Willis, reported that intellectual impairment was caused by abnormalities in the brain. Prior to the 18th century, individuals with intellectual disabilities were typically cared for by families and religious institutions. During the 1700s and 1800s, it became less common for care of individuals with intellectual challenges to be provided by families, and these individuals were often housed in large institutions instead. These individuals also became increasingly devalued by society, as evidenced by the eugenics movement in the early 20th century. In 1905 Alfred Binet created the first standardized test for measuring intelligence, and by the 1950's children with developmental disabilities were being provided with educational services (Wehmeyer, 2013).

During the late 1960s through the 1970s some states began to discontinue the segregation of individuals with intellectual disabilities in large institutions, associated with movements such as "Normalization" and "Deinstitutionalization." In 1965 Burton Blatt and photographer Fred Kaplan photographed the inhuman conditions that existed in institutions in the United States. The photos were published in the iconic book *Christmas in Purgatory. A Photographic Essay on Mental Retardation* in 1970 (Blatt & Kaplan, 1970). In 1969 psychologist Wolf Wolfensberger published *The Origin and Nature of*

DOI: 10.4324/9781003639121-3

Our Institutional Models, which described society's treatment of individuals with disabilities as less than human. He proposed that all individuals have the capacity to make contributions to society and that individuals with intellectual and other disabilities should be provided with the same basic human rights as the rest of the population (Wolfensberger, 1969). Burton Blatt continued his pioneering efforts in this field with multiple publications, including *Exodus from Pandemonium. Human Abuse and a Reformation of Public Policy* (1970) and *Souls in Extremis* (1973). In 1980 the Civil Rights of Institutionalized Persons Act in the United States was passed, and during the 1980s and 1990s more information was provided to the public regarding the substandard conditions in many institutions. A movement to change to community-based methods of providing services emerged, and the majority of institutions were eventually closed (Wehmeyer, 2013).

TERMINOLOGY

The terminology used to describe individuals with intellectual disabilities has undergone many changes over the past two centuries, as certain "medical" labels came to be considered disparaging and derogatory. The American Association on Mental Retardation (AAMR) used the term "mental retardation," and this term was also included in previous editions of the American Psychiatric Association's *Diagnostic and Statistical Manual of Mental Disorders* (DSM). In 2006, AAMR was changed to the "American Association on Intellectual and Developmental Disabilities." In 2010, federal law 111–256, Rosa's Law, replaced the term mental retardation with intellectual disability (ID). The bill was introduced in the United Sates Senate by Barbara Mikulski (Committee on Health, Education, Labor and Pensions, 2010). The American Psychiatric Association (APA) also changed the diagnosis to "intellectual disability" in their fifth edition of the *Diagnostic and Statistical Manual of Mental Disorders* (DSM-5). The diagnosis is also referred to as "intellectual developmental disorder" (American Psychiatric Association, 2013; American Psychiatric Association, 2022). Please note that these two diagnostic labels will be used interchangeably throughout this book.

LEGAL PROGRESS

In addition to terminology and societal changes, multiple federal policy changes throughout the 20th and 21st centuries greatly affected the education of children with disabilities. Many of these laws and policies will continue to have relevance throughout this book.

During the 1950s and 1960s, the federal government began to recognize the importance of establishing programs and supports for individuals with disabilities. Federal laws were created to support the training of professionals with expertise in teaching and assisting children with developmental challenges and providing state support for educational programs. It is notable that because of the 10th Amendment of the U.S. Constitution, most educational policies have been decided at the state and local levels, and as a result, there has always been variability in educational programs and services from state to state.

The Rehabilitation Act of 1973 improved the availability of grants for state rehabilitation services and expanded research and training programs. It also made the Secretary of Health, Education, and Welfare responsible for coordination of programs designed for individuals with disabilities within the Department of Health, Education, and Welfare and created the Rehabilitation Services Administration. This Act prohibited federal government programs from discriminating based on an individual's disability, extended civil rights to people with disabilities, and provided educational and employment opportunities for children and adults with disabilities (Public Law 93–112, 87 Stat. 355, 1973).

On November 29, 1975, President Gerald Ford signed Public Law 94–142, the Education for All Handicapped Children Act (EHA) which guaranteed a free appropriate public education (FAPE) to children with disabilities in every U.S. state. This law provided special education services for children with disabilities, from 3 to 21 years of age, with assistance and financial incentives provided to the states. Before passage of the EHA, children with disabilities could be denied access to an educational program (Education for All Handicapped Children Act, 1975).

During the 1980s and 1990s there was an effort to expand opportunities for children with disabilities, including placement in the least restrictive educational environment. Efforts were made to have children with disabilities attend their neighborhood schools. The 1985 reauthorization (Public Law 99–457) of EHA mandated that states provide programs and services to children with special needs beginning at birth. This provided access to early intervention programs for qualified children from birth to three years of age.

In 1990, EHA was reauthorized in Congress, and the Act's name was changed to the Individuals with Disabilities Education Act (IDEA), replacing the label of "handicapped" with "disability." It also added traumatic brain injury and autism as disability categories. As a result of IDEA, public schools could not refuse to enroll students because of their disability, no matter how severe, the only exception being if a child had a transmissible disease. Accommodations for every child were required with the goal of students receiving their education in the least restrictive environment, therefore decreasing the risk of a child with a disability from being completely segregated from their peers.

As a result of EHA and IDEA, each child is required to be provided with an individualized education program (IEP) based on their specific educational needs. Working with education professionals and parents, the IEP, a legal written statement, describes how the child performs academically, what their ongoing goals are, performance markers, and what services and resources are needed to potentially achieve those goals. An IEP is reviewed and revised at least once a year by a team including educators, parents, students themselves from the age of 14, and others who have knowledge and/ or expertise needed for the development of the student's special education program. The IEP must contain measurable goals written for the coming year, and must be reviewed annually. An updated evaluation for a child who has an IEP is required every three years, or sooner if needed, and it must be conducted within 60 days of parental permission. The IEP has become a vital document for millions of students across the United States.

It is also important to note that as a result of the recognition of ethnic and socioeconomic imbalances in children who were receiving special education services, the 1997 reauthorization of IDEA included the mandate that diagnosing learning challenges should not be related to "cultural factors," "environmental or economic disadvantage," or being of "limited English proficiency." It also required that the analysis of special education data include ethnicity in order to assess the characteristics, systems, and methods that may result in disproportionate identification of children with special needs (Shifrer et al., 2011).

IEPs are designed for children beginning at three-years-old. Children who are younger than three and qualify for early intervention receive an individualized family service plan (IFSP). An IFSP is also a legal document that describes the needs of the infant or young child and the child's family in order to provide them with appropriate services.

Additional amendments to IDEA in the 1990's included providing transition services for adolescents in high school to adult living. Congress mandated that as a part of a student's IEP, an individual transition plan (ITP) must be developed to help the student transition to life as an adult. Reauthorization of IDEA during the 1990's also included improving students' access to the general education curriculum, giving states the opportunity to expand the age of children diagnosed with "developmental delay", and giving parents legal rights to resolve disputes with the school system through mediation.

The reauthorization of IDEA in 2004 aligned with the No Child Left Behind Act requirements; it expanded the criteria for access to early intervention (EI) services, included the requirement for improved account-ability from educational programs, and raised the standards for special educa-tion teachers. In August 2006, modifications to IDEA required schools to include evidenced-based interventions and specific evaluation criteria in the process for determining eligibility for special education services and provid-ing appropriate services for students with learning challenges. The 2006 regulations also addressed other new requirements included in the 2004 reauthorization, such as the resolution process required when a parent files a complaint, and the requirement to provide equitable services for paren-tally placed private school children with disabilities to the local educational agency (LEA) in which the private school is located. Additional clarifications were made to IDEA during the 21st century, including improving parental rights regarding a child's education and addressing the allocation of funds. The goal of revisions made in 2016 was to promote equity under IDEA. It also helped to prevent children with disabilities from being disproportion-ately removed from their educational placements for disciplinary reasons. As discussed previously, in 2010, Rosa's Law replaced references to "mental retardation" in the Federal law with "intellectual disability" or "intellectual disabilities." In 2017 the U.S. Department of Education published regula-tions based on Rosa's Law that also aligned with the Every Student Succeeds Act of 2015 (ESSA), ensuring language is consistent with the federal statute and improving access to a high-quality education for all students.

In summary, IDEA has provided students with disabilities a free, appro-priate public education; individualized education programs; education in the least restrictive environment; a requirement for schools to implement evaluation standards to determine qualification for special education ser-vices; participation of parents/legal guardians, students from the age of 14, and appropriate educators, therapists, and school professionals in the special educational process; and assurance of parental awareness regard-ing their rights and responsibilities and how disagreements are handled. The impact of IDEA was far reaching in expanding educational rights for children with disabilities and continues to keep those regulations at the forefront of educational practices.

For the sake of completion, it is also important to include three additional historic federal laws that were designed to protect the rights of individuals with disabilities: Section 504 of the Rehabilitation Act of 1973, the Ameri-cans with Disabilities Act (ADA) of 1990, and the revised ADA of 2008. Section 504 of the Rehabilitation Act of 1973 was a federal law designed to protect the rights of individuals with physical, cognitive, or mental health disability. Today, a 504 accommodation plan may be implemented at school for a child who does not qualify for an IEP but has a diagnosis and/or chal-lenge that requires accommodations and supports – for example, a diagnosis of attention–deficit/hyperactivity disorder (ADHD) alone will often not qualify a child for an IEP but will likely qualify the child for a 504 Accommodation Plan. (Wright & Wright 2023).

Now that the history lesson has been completed, let us meet some children whose parents express concerns about their development.

CASE STUDIES

Ethan walked on time but was delayed in his speech development. His parents were told by relatives that boys are not as verbal as girls. At his two-year well child care visit with his pediatrician, it was brought to their attention that he should be speaking in phrases; at that time Ethan was only saying "Mamma," "Dada," and "Baba." Ethan was referred for an early intervention evaluation, and his parents were informed that in addition to his speech delays, he was also showing delays in other areas – for example, he did not follow simple directions, and he did not stack cubes or place pegs into a pegboard. Ethan's play that was observed included putting cubes into a container and dumping them out; banging objects together; and shaking a rattle in imitation. Ethan was diagnosed with global developmental delay. Ethan's parents wanted to know if Ethan's skills would eventually "catch up" to children his age, or if his presentation indicated that he had an intellectual disability.

Amelia appeared to be shy. She reached milestones on time with the exception of her speech. She was able to follow directions, but when she tried to speak, her parents reported that she would look at them and vocalize sounds rather than words. She also pointed and gestured in an attempt to try to tell others what she wanted but did not use words that they could understand. Amelia began preschool when she was three years old. She engaged in many preschool activities but continued to experience difficulties expressing herself. Amelia's teacher told her parents that Amelia would benefit from having an evaluation completed by the public-school special education team.

Isabella was born three months early. Her parents were informed that Isabella's prematurity placed her at risk for developmental delays. Isabella was tested by early intervention and they reported that she was between two and five months behind in her skills. She received early intervention services once a month. By the time Isabella was two-and-a-half years old, she had made a great deal of progress, but her parents continued to worry about Isabella's future. Would she continue to be considered developmentally delayed when she began attending school? Would she be diagnosed with an intellectual disability?

All children do not necessarily master developmental skills at exactly the same time. As described in Chapter 1, there is an age range during which it is considered typical for a child to achieve skills. Children who are not meeting developmental skills during the expected age range are considered "delayed" in these skills. Some children with developmental delays, but not all of them, may later be diagnosed with an ID.

DIAGNOSING A CHILD WITH AN INTELLECTUAL DISABILITY

The diagnosis of an ID, also referred to as intellectual developmental disorder, is a diagnosis made during childhood based on the results of standardized testing. Such testing historically included a child's Intelligence Quotient (IQ) and their Adaptive Functioning, that is, their ability to adapt to the demands of daily life (American Psychiatric Association, 2013; Morrison, 2014). Intelligence involves a thorough picture of an individual's cognitive functioning, which includes one's ability to problem solve, reason, think abstractly, and comprehend ideas and verbal information; the efficiency of an individual's learning; and one's ability to learn from experiences (American Association on Intellectual Developmental Disabilities [AAIDD], 2010). The diagnosis of an ID was traditionally defined by an IQ less than 70 as well as deficits in two or more adaptive behaviors. Although the DSM-5 no longer specified IQ scores as a diagnostic criterion, it continued to endorse that the functioning of individuals with an ID is two or more standard deviations below the mean of the general population. Adaptive functioning incorporates three areas: "conceptual", which includes cognitive-related areas such as language and problem solving; "social", which includes the ability to understand the experiences of others; and "practical", which includes managing and organizing personal issues and recreational activities. More importance was placed on adaptive functioning, including the ability to perform basic life skills (American Psychiatric Association, 2013; Morrison, 2014).

Despite modifications in criteria, the diagnosis of an ID is still not typically a definitive diagnosis until a child is old enough for standardized IQ and adaptive functioning testing to be completed by a psychologist (American Psychiatric Association, 2013; Morrison, 2014). A child who presents with delays in their skills, but is too young for standardized IQ and adaptive skill testing, may or may not be later diagnosed with an ID (Boat & Wu, 2015). At younger ages, a child's skills can fluctuate and/or appear more or less advanced based on many factors such as their interests, experiences, exposure to early learning, etc. Therefore, standardized testing and diagnostic conclusions most often occur when the child is school-aged or later.

Both the American Association on Intellectual and Developmental Disabilities and the DSM-5 classify ID by severity as "mild", "moderate", severe", and "profound." Previous categorization was based on IQ range in combination with standardized adaptive functioning scores, but more recently the focus has been on the level of support an individual requires in completion of daily living skills. Similar to the bell-shaped curve used to visualize population IQs (mean 100, standard deviation 15), the majority of individuals with ID fall into the mild range. These individuals can typically function in society with only minimal need for support. Individuals with moderate ID are typically able to take care of themselves and learn basic skills related to health and safety. Individuals with severe ID require supervision in many social situations and cannot typically live safely independently. Individuals with profound ID are unable to live independently and require close supervision and assistance with self-care. All levels of ID may be associated with other medical diagnoses, including genetic syndromes. However, as the level of severity of ID increases, so does the risk of additional medical diagnoses and problems (Boat & Wu, 2015). It is important to note that in addition to a child's level of ID severity, there are also other factors that contribute to a child's future ability to function successfully. Factors such as support systems, environmental modifications, social skills, medical issues, etc., can all have an impact on a child's ability to function as independently as possible.

In determining which standardized test to use, psychologists need to take into account whether there are factors that may affect a child's performance, such as motor, sensory, or communication challenges. Some current standardized intelligence tests for children include the Wechsler Intelligence Scale for Children (WISC; currently 5th edition) (Wechsler, 2014), the Stanford-Binet (Roid 2003), and the Kaufman Assessment Battery for Children (Kaufman & Kaufman, 2004). Each of these tests include several subtests in order to evaluate specific areas of a child's ability – for example, the child's verbal skills, working memory, nonverbal skills, fluid reasoning, crystallized thinking, etc. The minimum age for the WISC is six years old, the Kaufman Assessment Battery for Children is three years old, and the Stanford Binet is two years old. However, intelligence testing is typically considered more reliable and predictive beginning at about six years old. Of note, the Wechsler Preschool and Primary Scale of Intelligence was designed for younger children, ages two-and-a-half to seven. The Bayley Scales of Infant and Toddler Development (currently 4th edition) can assess the skills of infants and toddlers from 16 days to 42 months old. These tests provide a picture of a child's current strengths and weaknesses. Although the idea of an IQ is expected to be relatively stable over time, the younger a child is at the time of the assessment, the less one should be encouraged to make a prediction regarding future intelligence. As a general rule, the greater the severity of a young child's delays, the greater the risk that the child may eventually be diagnosed with an ID. Conversely, a child who has been diagnosed with mild ID may not have appeared to be significantly delayed when they were younger. There are two demographics worth noting regarding the diagnosis of ID: boys are more likely to be diagnosed with ID than girls, and poverty is a risk factor, particularly for mild ID (Boat & Wu, 2015).

Will a Child with Delays in Their Developmental Skills "Catch Up"?

It is not uncommon to hear stories about children who were delayed but eventually "caught up" to their peers and no longer had any developmental problems. It can be challenging to predict whether a child's skills will catch up. It may be that several family members presented similarly – for example, many individuals in the family did not begin walking until they were 18 or 19 months old, or were "late talkers" – but then went on to participate successfully in age-appropriate activities and did well at school. As stated above, the more significant the delays, the higher the risk for being diagnosed with an ID. Regardless of whether a child's skills may later "catch up" to their peers, infants and children who are younger than three years old who appear to be delayed in their skills can be evaluated by an early intervention program to determine if they qualify for assistance/intervention.

Other Diagnoses Associated with Developmental Delays in Children

Some children achieve skills later than their peers but similar to the ages of siblings and other family members. Like their siblings, they may later be assessed and demonstrate age-appropriate skills.

Some children may lack specific opportunities that may result in mild delays in one or more of their skills. For example, a limited amount of safe space available for a child to move independently, with the child being held by an adult or placed in a "jumper" for multiple hours each day, has the potential to be associated with some delays in the achievement of motor skills.

Some children who are delayed in their developmental skills may later be tested and have an IQ above 70. Some of these children will have presented with language delays that affected other areas of their development, and the possibility that they may have been presenting with an intellectual developmental disorder may have previously been considered.

A child with a hearing impairment typically presents with communication challenges, and children with vision challenges can present with delays in fine and gross motor skills. **It is important for any child who presents with delays in their skills to have their hearing and vision assessed.**

Children with a specific learning disability can present with delays in their skills, but their delays are typically specific to certain areas – for example, an IQ greater than 70, but certain academic achievement scores under 70.

Children with autism spectrum disorder can meet criteria for an ID, but there are also individuals with autism spectrum disorder whose IQ and adaptive functioning are not below average.

Children who are born premature are at risk for developmental challenges. However, if they are performing skills that are appropriate for their corrected age, the concern decreases. A child's corrected age is typically used to assess the appropriateness of their developmental skills, until the child is about two years old.

Let us return to Ethan, Amelia, and Isabella.

CASE STUDIES

Ethan received early intervention services. He made improvements in all of his skills but continued to demonstrate skills more similar to a younger child. He qualified for an IEP in preschool and elementary school. During elementary school results of standardized IQ testing revealed a verbal IQ of 65 and a nonverbal IQ of 68, with similar standard scores on adaptive functioning testing. Ethan was diagnosed with a mild intellectual disability.

Amelia had testing completed by the special education team. All of her standard scores were within the average range except for her expressive language. She was referred for a hearing assessment and was tested to have normal hearing. She was diagnosed with an expressive language disorder and received speech-language therapy twice a week during preschool and elementary school. Of note, during elementary school, Amelia also required some assistance with English Language Arts (ELA) subjects.

Isabella received early intervention services. Even though her testing results showed that she continued to be a little behind for her chronological age, her skills were appropriate for a child who was three months younger; that is, her skills were appropriate for her "corrected age." Isabella did not qualify for participation in an inclusion preschool program based on testing completed by the public schools before she turned three. She attended a traditional preschool and did well in elementary school.

CAUSES OF ID

There are multiple known causes of ID but children can also be diagnosed with ID without a known etiology/cause.

Known causes include genetic diagnosis such as chromosomal abnormalities (for example, trisomy 21/Down syndrome), recessive and dominant genetic disorders (for example, Fragile X syndrome, velo-cardio-facial syndrome, neurofibromatosis), and inborn errors of metabolism (for example, Phenylketonuria [PKU]). Some genetic diagnoses are inherited from one or both parents and some occur spontaneously ("de novo"). Genetic disorders can have physical features and sometimes medical problems associated with the diagnoses. In addition, genetic, metabolic, and endocrine disorders that are treatable (i.e., treatment can prevent a child from developing an intellectual disability) are typically screened for immediately after birth – for example, thyroid abnormalities, PKU, and other inborn errors of metabolism.

There are also issues that can occur during a pregnancy that may increase a child's risk for ID, including alcohol use, fetal malnutrition, trauma, certain maternal infections, and placental and other anatomic abnormalities. After birth, exposure to toxins such as lead, certain infections such as bacterial meningitis, and central nervous system trauma can increase a child's risk of being diagnosed with an ID.

BEHAVIORS AND OTHER ISSUES THAT CAN BE OBSERVED AT HIGHER FREQUENCY IN CHILDREN WITH ID

Individuals who have been diagnosed with an ID are at increased risk for other diagnoses that can sometimes be related to central nervous system/brain abnormalities. This includes an increased risk for behavioral challenges, sleep problems, motor/movement problems, seizures, and abnormal growth patterns. However, not all children with an ID will experience these types of issues. It is also important to note that although a diagnosis of ID can increase a child's risk of behavioral issues, one must remember that a child's behavior is often commensurate with their intellectual/developmental level. For example, if an eight-year-old child's intelligence and adaptive functioning testing places them at the level of a two year old, their behavior is more likely to be similar to that of a two year old.

TREATMENT WITH MEDICATION

There are no medications that directly improve an individual's intelligence. However, similar to children who have no cognitive challenges, children with IDs who have additional diagnoses such as ADHD can often benefit from treatment with medication.

INTERVENTIONS AND SUPPORTS FOR CHILDREN WITH ID

Classroom supports for children with IDs can vary from state to state. In addition, specific supports may vary depending on the severity of a child's disability and any additional challenges that they may present with – for example, additional diagnosis such as ADHD or other behavioral disorders. A child with an ID will likely benefit from a relatively smaller classroom size where they can receive small group and possibly individualized instruction. Their academic curriculum will likely need to be modified. If a child's disability negatively impacts their ability to complete activities of daily living (for example, self-care) then this would be appropriate to add to their educational program. Moreover, if a child's disability results in limited reading and math skills, gearing their program in upper grades to functional academics – reading signs, managing money – and exploring supervised vocational opportunities in the community would be beneficial. A child with an ID may have attentional skills similar to a younger child, therefore many of the modifications for children with ADHD may also be helpful – for example, clearly specifying rules and instructions; providing frequent opportunities for supervision and teacher feedback; and making sure instructions are given in relatively brief and understandable sentences. Providing visual examples for children such as number lines and alphabet tape can also provide assistance.

Similar to typical children, children with intellectual developmental disorders benefit from structure both at school and at home.

AUTHORS' COMMENTARY

Although the goal for a child is placement in an educational setting in the least restrictive environment, optimally with typical children, there are some children with ID who require a more intensive educational setting, particularly if they present with significant behavioral challenges. A collaborative approach between parents and the special education team is essential in order to explore the most optimal educational environment for each child. In our experience, we have observed some schools that offer only inclusive classroom settings, with their school district being able to offer the supports each child needs within the inclusive setting. Other schools do not have the resources needed to enable a child with intensive special needs to be successful in an inclusion classroom. However, even with the ability to offer optimal services within an inclusive setting, some children may still require at least part of their day in a smaller, more therapeutic environment in order to provide them with a successful educational experience.

Discussions with parents should include encouraging them to attempt to adapt their expectations according to their child's cognitive level and developmental skills. As children mature, discussions regarding a child's future should be gradually incorporated into the parents' interactions with support professionals, particularly the special education team. Topics should include post-secondary education and adult programs, qualifications for social security income, the amount of supervision an adolescent will likely need during adulthood, and legal issues such as guardianship.

CASE STUDIES

Ethan continued to receive special education services. During high school he was provided with some supervised experiences in the community. He was friendly and a hard worker and was offered a paid job in an office where he received supervision. The job was initially part of his educational program, which continued through his early 20's. The office later hired him as a permanent employee.

Final note: Although impairments in functioning associated with ID are generally predicted to continue through adulthood, appropriate supports can often enable individuals with ID to function well within society (Boat & Wu, 2015). Therefore, an important goal for professionals who care for children is to provide the supports and assistance children need in order for them to achieve their maximum potential.

HANDOUT FOR CAREGIVERS

Intellectual Developmental Disorder/ Intellectual Disability (ID)

This diagnosis is based on standardized testing of cognitive and adaptive functioning completed by a psychologist, together with information about the level of support a child requires in order to complete daily living skills. A definitive diagnosis of ID is typically not made until early elementary school. Infants and young children who are diagnosed with delays in their developmental skills, may or may not be later diagnosed with an intellectual developmental disorder.

Common Questions

How Can I Help My Child?

Try to make your expectations for your child appropriate for their cognitive/intellectual level. If an elementary school child's cognitive ability is more similar to a preschool level, then expectations of their behavior and attention should be at that same level.

Provide a structured environment and create a schedule – i.e., specific time periods for waking up, bedtime, chores, homework, playtime, TV time, meals, etc. Explain any changes in routine ahead of time so that the child understands and can anticipate the changes.

Give instructions as simply and clearly as possible, demonstrating if necessary. Ask your child to repeat them back to you, then praise them when they respond correctly. Do not give more than one or two instructions at one time. If a task is difficult, break it into smaller parts and teach each part separately.

Think about the experience of learning something challenging – that is likely what your child faces when attempting to learn things that may come more easily to typical children. Teaching a child with an ID requires patience. It is often helpful to break down information into smaller, simpler steps. Repetition is important for all learning, and visual cues are often helpful.

Try to work as a partner with your child's special education team. Try to educate yourself regarding special education policies and procedures. Engaging in parent groups can also often provide you with support and information.

Can My Child's intelligence quotient (IQ) Change?

Although an individual's intelligence quotient is theoretically stable, since a child's development is continually changing with maturity, there can

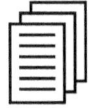

sometimes be some variability in a child's testing scores over time. This is particularly true when the initial testing is completed at a young age. However, it is notable that if there is a clear downward trend in a child's intelligence test scores, medical testing to explore diagnoses that are associated with a decline in intellectual functioning is typically indicated.

Will My Child Ever Be Completely Independent?

The ability of an individual with intellectual disabilities to become a completely independent adult can be dependent upon multiple factors, including the level of a child's ID – adults with mild levels of ID can often live independently. In addition, mental health and behavioral challenges can have a negative impact on an individual's ability to function completely independently.

Teaching children and adolescents with intellectual disabilities life skills as part of their educational programs and at home, while also providing them with gradual, cautious independence at home, can have a positive impact on their ability to function independently as an adult.

BIBLIOGRAPHY

American Association of Intellectual and Developmental Disorders (AAIDD). https://www.aaidd.org.

American Association on Intellectual Developmental Disabilities (AAIDD) (2010). *Intellectual disability: Definition, classification, and systems of supports.* Washington, DC: AAIDD.

American Psychiatric Association (APA) (2013). *Diagnostic and Statistical Manual of Mental Disorders – 5th edition.* Arlington, VA: American Psychiatric Association Publishing.

American Psychiatric Association (APA) (2022). *Diagnostic and Statistical Manual of Mental Disorders – 5th edition. Text Revision (DSM-5-TR).* Arlington, VA: American Psychiatric Association Publishing.

The Americans with Disabilities Act (ADA). https://www.ada.gov.

The Arc. https://www.thearc.org.

Bayley, N. (2006). *The Bayley Scales of Infant and Toddler Development – 4th edition.* San Antonio, Texas: Harcourt Assessment.

Blatt, B. (1970). *Exodus from Pandemonium. Human Abuse and Reformation of Public policy.* Boston, MA: Allyn and Bacon.

Blatt, B. (1973) *Souls in Extremis.* Boston, MA: Allyn and Bacon.

Blatt, B., & Kaplan F. (1970). *Christmas in purgatory. A photographic essay on mental retardation.* Boston, MA: Allyn and Bacon.

Boat, T. F., & Wu, J. T. (Eds); Committee to Evaluate the Supplemental Security Income Disability Program for Children with Mental Disorders; Board on the Health of Select Populations; Board on Children, Youth, and Families; Institute of Medicine; Division of Behavioral and Social Sciences and Education; The National Academies of Sciences, Engineering, and Medicine. (2015) Clinical characteristics of intellectual disabilities. In *Mental Disorders and Disabilities Among Low Income Children.* Washington, DC: National Academies Press. Available from: https://www.ncbi.nlm.nih.gov/books/NBK332877/.

Chan, J. (2024). Rights of persons with disabilities: Current status and future directions. *Advances in Neurodevelopmental Disorders.* https://doi.org/10.1007/s41252-024-00392-3.

Committee on Health, Education, Labor and Pensions (2010). Public Law 111–256. 111th Congress. Congressional Record: Vol 156.

Education for All Handicapped Children Act (1975, June 2). S.6, Public Law 94–142. 94th Congress: 1st Session. Report No. 94–168.

Individuals with Disabilities Education Act (IDEA) (2004). 20 U.S.C. Section 1400.

Kaufman, A. S., & Kaufman, N. L. (2004). *The Kaufman Assessment Battery for Children – 2nd edition.* Circle Pines, MN: American Guidance Service.

Morrison J. (2014). *DSM-5 Made Easy: The Clinician's Guide to Diagnosis.* New York, NY: Guilford Press.

Rehabilitation Act of 1973. Public Law 93–112, 87 Stat. 355.

Roid, G. H. (2003). *Stanford-Binet Intelligence Scales – 5th edition.* Itasca, IL: Riverside Publishing.

Shifrer, D., Muller, C., & Callahan, R. (2011) Disproportionality and learning disabilities: Parsing apart race, socioeconomic status, and language. *Journal of Leaning Disabilities,* 44(3): 246–257. https://doi.org/10.1177/0022219410374236.

U.S. Department of Education. https://www.ed.gov.

Wechsler, D. (2014) *WISC-V: Wechsler Intelligence Scale for Children – 5th edition.* Bloomington, MN: Pearson.

Wehmeyer, M. L. (2013). *The Story of Intellectual Disability: An Evolution of Meaning, Understanding, and Public Perception.* Baltimore, Maryland: Brookes Publishing.

Wolfensberger, W. (1969). *The Origin and Nature of Our Institutional Models.* Washington, D.C.: President's Committee on Mental Retardation.

Wright, P. W. D., & Wright, P. D. (2023) *Wrights Law: Special Education Law – 3rd edition.* Hartfield, VA: Harbor House Law Press Inc.

CHAPTER 4

Autism Spectrum or Just a Little Different?

When I (Jo-Ann Bier) was training as a special education teacher in the 1970's, the diagnosis of autism was less common than it is today. After transitioning into the medical field, I began to observe an increase in caregiver concerns regarding this diagnosis. The number of children diagnosed with autism has spiked even more over the last few decades. What is the reason for this increase? Is it a result of an increase in awareness of the diagnosis? A change in the definition associated with an expansion of the criteria to include a wide "spectrum" of children? A need for a specific diagnosis in order for a child to receive supports and services? We would suggest that the answer is "all of the above," as well as possible additional factors that have together contributed to the current increase in the number of children diagnosed with autism. The diagnosis currently encompasses a large spectrum of children and has become a frequent subject of television shows, movies, and countless articles and books. As a result, professionals who care for children and their families are likely to frequently hear parents and other caregivers question whether their child may be presenting with behaviors suggestive of autism spectrum disorder (ASD) – sometimes based on their own observations and sometimes based on concerns expressed by well-meaning friends and relatives. Of course, this can present parents with uncertainty and stress. In addition, sometimes professionals offer different opinions, which can add to a parent's confusion. And then, as if to further complicate the questions families face, sometimes parents hear that intervention might help even if their child does not appear to meet criteria for a diagnosis of ASD. No wonder parents get overwhelmed! This chapter focuses on features of the diagnosis of ASD and state of the art treatments and therapies. The idea that some of these features can be observed in typically developing children and children with other diagnoses will also be discussed.

DOI: 10.4324/9781003639121-4

Let us meet three children described here by their parents.

CASE STUDIES

Olivia's language skills were delayed. Her older sister, on the other hand, was extremely verbal. Olivia's mother initially thought that Olivia was not talking because her sister was speaking and interpreting for her. But when Olivia was still not saying any words at two years old, she became concerned. She also noticed that Olivia sometimes covered her ears with her hands in response to the vacuum cleaner and other loud noises. Her neighbor suggested that Olivia should be evaluated for autism.

Liam is three years old. His aunt noticed some behaviors that she felt may be concerning: Liam has always loved cars and trucks. He likes to line up his toy vehicles, which is one of the only times she saw him stay still. He can get agitated and even have a complete "melt down" if someone interferes with his methodical lining up of his cars. Liam's aunt brought up her concerns with Liam's parents. Is his behavior a sign of autism? Is Liam just really into cars? Liam's mom didn't know how to respond. She did some of her own research but found an overwhelming amount of information that was difficult to decipher. Is Liam showing signs of autism spectrum? Liam's mother began to feel stressed by the contrasting opinions she heard, so she came to you for assistance.

Noah's parents could not have been more excited when Noah was born. He was his parents' first-born child, and there were no problems during or after his delivery. As an infant, Noah hated being put on his belly and cried during "tummy time." He said, "dadada" when he was almost one year old, but it was not clear if he meant "daddy" when he said this – he just seemed to say it randomly. Noah responded to music, and just after he turned one he began "singing" some repetitive pieces of songs – for example, "e-i-e-i-o." Then, when he was about 14 months old, he started vocalizing less. He stopped making as many sounds. He even stopped singing. Relatives informed Noah's parents that boys do not talk as early as girls, so at first, they were not too concerned. Then, at his 18-month pediatrician appointment, Noah's doctor reported that he should be saying multiple words. She also reported that Noah's tendency to focus on the wheels of his toy cars, watching them spin, and his sensitivities to certain food textures and colors and certain noises appeared concerning. His pediatrician referred Noah to early intervention. That was the first time his parents heard the word "autism" mentioned.

Do some of these behaviors sound familiar? Are these children present-ing with personality quirks? Are any of these children autistic? Which ones? Let us try to sort out this currently relatively common, but fairly complicated, diagnosis.

AUTISM SPECTRUM DISORDER (ASD)

In the 2013 fifth edition of the *Diagnostic and Statistical Manual* (DSM-5), the diagnosis of autistic disorder/autism was grouped with some previously separate diagnoses, including pervasive developmental disorder (PDD) and Asperger syndrome, under the single diagnosis of autism spectrum dis-order (ASD) (American Psychiatric Association, 2013; Morrison, 2014). Although some diagnostic evaluation tools (for example, the Autism Diagnostic Observation Schedule [ADOS] [Lord et al., 2012]) differenti-ate between a diagnosis of autism and of ASD, these labels are often used interchangeably in the public. Professionals determining whether or not a child meets criteria for ASD review the child's history, including reports by caregivers, and also assess the child's developmental and behavioral pres-entation. Specifically, they look for problems in the areas of social interac-tion, social communication, and certain behavioral patterns the child may exhibit.

Children with ASD demonstrate deficiencies in social interaction and social communication. For example, these children may appear discon-nected from other people and appear to show a lack of interest in other people, including their peers. Specific characteristics of ASD can include limited eye contact and a lack of responsiveness to their name (after they have reached the developmental level when this would be expected). Children with ASD demonstrate communication that appears unusual or "atypical" – for example, they may use language from movies and televi-sion shows, i.e., "scripted" language, use language out of context, repeat or echo phrases that were previously heard out of context, and misuse pro-nouns. In addition to lack of age-appropriate and unusual/atypical verbal language, children with ASD also demonstrate a weakness in their non-verbal communication. For example, they may not point to the refrigera-tor as a request for something to eat or drink, or hold their hands up and look at an adult indicating the desire to be picked up. Conventional ges-tures, such as waving hello or good-bye, shrugging one's shoulders, or put-ting a hand up with palm facing out to indicate stop, are often absent from the child's repertoire of behavioral interactions with others. Children with ASD often lack the behavior of showing something to another individual in an attempt to share the object or experience with the other individual, i.e, demonstrate "joint attention." Even if a child with ASD is verbal, they may demonstrate an unusually strong preference for talking only about a specific topic in a "one-way" conversation, with a decreased interest when someone else tries to engage them in conversation (American Psychiatric Association, 2013; Bridgemohan et al., 2019; Morrison, 2014).

In addition to weaknesses in social communication, children with ASD demonstrate unusual/atypical behaviors, which can include repetitive movements; inflexibility regarding changes of routine; intense interests in very specific areas or activities; and unusual sensitivities and/or seeking out of sensory (hearing, touch, vision) experiences. Examples of some specific behaviors that may be observed include self-stimulatory behaviors/motor stereotypies – for example, hand flapping, finger flicking, spinning objects, or turning continuously; using the same phrases repeatedly and out of context; spinning wheels on toy vehicles continuously; and spinning or flipping puzzle pieces continuously, rather than using them appropriately. Although most children prefer a routine, a child with ASD can be strongly insistent on specific routines, with any change in routine sometimes resulting in a severe "meltdown" or outburst. Finally, sensory issues may include abnormal sensitivity ("hypersensitivity") to noises, clothing, or food tastes or textures, or seeking out of sensory experiences ("hyposensitivity") such as "crashing" into things, a need for movement, or a preference for spicy or crunchy types of foods (American Psychiatric Association, 2013; Bridgemohan et al., 2019; Morrison, 2014).

All of these behaviors offer important clues. Children with autism can display some or all of them. It is important to note that sometimes children who do not have autism, but who might have other developmental problems and/or delays, also exhibit some of these behaviors. Moreover, typically developing children can sometimes be observed to demonstrate some of these behaviors as well. The presentation of unusual or atypical behaviors alone does not automatically indicate an ASD diagnosis. A comprehensive evaluation that involves consideration of all the above-mentioned factors and criteria must be completed by a qualified medical professional to determine whether or not a diagnosis of ASD is appropriate for the child.

CASE STUDIES

Olivia and **Noah** exhibited delays in their language skills. Noah also seemed to demonstrate a regression (loss of skills) in his language. Olivia is highly sensitive to noise. **Liam** has a preference for lining up his toy vehicles, and becomes upset when this behavior is interrupted. None of these behaviors, taken individually, definitively indicate ASD. While each of these characteristics can be seen in children with ASD, they can also appear in children who have other developmental problems and/or delays and even some children whose developmental course may later be determined to be age-appropriate. But these children's behaviors offer important clues, indicating that careful, professional evaluation is needed.

DIAGNOSING A CHILD WITH ASD

Although there has been recent exploration of biomarkers to assist in identifying risk factors for the diagnosis of ASD, there is no specific medical test that can definitively diagnose a child with ASD. (It is worth mentioning, however, that medical studies/tests may be recommended to search for possible underlying causes if a child is diagnosed with ASD.) Children who are not ultimately determined to meet criteria for ASD do sometimes exhibit features of this diagnosis – for example, sensory sensitivities, compulsions, or social awkwardness. If these issues do not have a significant negative impact on how a child is functioning at school, home, and in other settings, then a diagnosis of ASD is less likely.

Some primary care physicians, teachers, and counselors are comfortable using the DSM criteria to make an initial diagnosis of ASD, including administering questionnaires and possibly some screening tests. However, a definitive diagnosis is typically confirmed by professionals with specific expertise in making this diagnosis – for example, a developmental-behavioral pediatrician, psychologist, neurodevelopmental pediatrician, psychiatrist, or neurologist. The diagnosis of ASD is a clinical diagnosis, drawing on information provided by parents, teachers, and early intervention staff, together with observations of the child. Evaluation of a child's communication and cognitive skills should be included in the assessment. Tools to assess behavior such as the Behavior Assessment System for Children (Bradstreet et al., 2017) and the Child Behavior Checklist (Havdahl et al., 2016) are not specifically designed to diagnose ASD, but their results may indicate some features of this diagnosis (Hyman et al., 2020). As part of the ASD assessment, specific standardized questionnaires may be used – for example, the Childhood Autism Rating Scale (CARS) 2nd edition; the Social Communication Questionnaire; the Social Responsiveness Scale (Parent & Teacher), and the Autism Diagnostic Interview (revised) (Constantino et al., 2003; Corsello et al., 2007; Hyman et al., 2020; Rutter et al., 2003). The Autism Diagnostic Observation Schedule (ADOS) 2nd edition is a semi-structured interview and play observation tool designed to assess children's social communication and behavior. Modules are used based on a child's age and communication skills, and the child is assessed during structured play schemes – for example, a pretend birthday party or bubble play, and other reciprocal play activities (Lord et al., 2012). Although the ADOS has sometimes been referred to as the "gold standard" for diagnosing ASD, recent studies have shown that this evaluation tool, although beneficial, may not be necessary in making the diagnosis. Results of a prospective 2019–2020 study completed by Barbaresi and colleagues revealed that diagnoses of ASD made by developmental-behavioral pediatricians with vs. without the ADOS were consistent in 90.0% of cases. The study therefore suggested that completion of the ADOS is not a requirement in order to make an initial diagnosis of ASD; it was also reported that developmental-behavioral pediatricians could identify which children would benefit from having the ADOS completed (Barbaresi et al., 2022). It is important to reiterate, however, that the diagnosis of ASD should only be made after a comprehensive evaluation that combines a thorough history, examination, and completion of standardized surveys and/or tests by a professional with expertise in the diagnosis.

Since the diagnosis of ASD is not based on a specific laboratory or other medical test and is based at least partially on a professional's clinical judgment, professionals do not always agree about whether a child meets full criteria for autism. A single observation of a child may not give a medical professional enough information to make a determination. One doctor's visit provides only a snapshot of a child. Sometimes children are tired or ill and demonstrate behaviors that are not typical for them on their evaluation day. Seeing a child on multiple occasions and getting input from others such as therapists, parents, grandparents, and teachers can be beneficial.

It is also important to remember that children can and do change over time. They may behave differently as they mature and develop new skills. This new level of maturity and skill development can allow a child to show skills that were not evident during an earlier appointment. It has been reported that about 9% of children who are diagnosed with ASD in early childhood may no longer meet criteria for ASD by young adulthood. Data have indicated that these children who ultimately "outgrow" this diagnosis are more likely to have stronger cognitive skills, received early intervention, and demonstrated a decrease in stereotypies over time (Hyman et al., 2020). Some children also later transition to alternative diagnoses (for example, obsessive-compulsive disorder [OCD], anxiety disorder, attention-deficit/ hyperactivity disorder [ADHD]). Although cognitive and language skills during childhood are related to outcome, it has also been reported that the quality of life during adulthood in individuals with high functioning ASD is related to community and family supports (Hyman et al., 2020). It is therefore important to implement a "team approach" in ASD management – therapists, teachers, physicians, social workers, and counselors all contribute to improving a child and family's quality of life while navigating the complexities of this increasingly common diagnosis.

PREVALENCE AND DEMOGRAPHICS

An increase in the prevalence of ASD has been observed over time. The Autism and Developmental Disabilities Monitoring (ADDM) Network was created in 2000 to provide information regarding the prevalence of children who have been diagnosed with ASD across several U.S. states, based on an ASD evaluation, special education classification, or an international classification of diseases (ICD) code.

Data from 2010 reported a lower prevalence rate for the diagnosis of ASD in four-year-old children vs. eight-year-old children, but a higher proportion of four-year-old children diagnosed with both ASD and an intellectual disability (ID). The report from the American Academy of Pediatrics (AAP) Council on Children with Disabilities, Section on Developmental and Behavioral Pediatric suggested that this may be related to a later diagnosis of ASD in children with average intellectual abilities. They cite data indicating that a later age in diagnosis is associated with milder presentations (Hyman et al., 2020).

In 2020, it was reported that the prevalence of ASD in eight-year-old children across 11 states within the ADDM Network was one in 36 children. These estimates were reported to be higher than previous ADDM Network estimates. ASD has consistently been reported to be diagnosed more frequently in boys, with the 2020 data reporting a prevalence of 43 per 1000 for boys and 11.4 per 1000 for girls. 2020 data were notable for some changes in racial demographics. The diagnosis of ASD was previously more commonly reported in White children, but in 2020 it was reported that the prevalence of ASD was lower among eight-year-old White children than among other racial and ethnic groups. Reported prevalence data per 1000 children included the following: non-Hispanic Asian or Pacific Islander children 33.4; Hispanic children 31.6; non-Hispanic Black or African American children 29.3; non-Hispanic Native American or Alaska Native children 26.5; non-Hispanic White children 24.3; children of two or more races 22.9. Children with ID had earlier ages of ASD diagnosis (43 months) than those without a diagnosis of ID (53 months). An increased ASD prevalence was associated with lower household income at three of the 11 sites. Moreover, there were overall prevalence rate differences among the network sites, including a prevalence of 23.3 per 1,000 eight-year-old children reported in Maryland vs. 44.9 per 1,000 in California (Maenner et al. 2023).

Why has the number of children diagnosed with ASD increased? We feel that the answer may be related to many factors. An increased awareness of the diagnosis of autism has likely increased the number of children suspected of being autistic. In addition, the definition and criteria for autism has changed over time, so it would make sense that the number of children diagnosed with autism/now ASD would also change. For example, some children previously did not meet criteria for autism but met criteria for Asperger syndrome or Pervasive Developmental Disorder/Delay–Not Otherwise Specified (PDD–NOS), but in 2013 the characteristics of these diagnoses were categorized under the umbrella of "autism spectrum disorders." Many of the children with Asperger and PDD therefore transitioned to a diagnosis of autism spectrum disorder. The reason for the change and variability in racial and geographic demographics reported in 2020 requires further investigation. We feel that attempting to maximize optimal services and supports for children and families in all demographic areas, ethnicities, and financial means needs to be a priority.

Now let us return to Olivia, Liam, and Noah.

CASE STUDIES

Olivia and **Noah** exhibited delays in their language skills, Olivia was sensitive to loud noises and **Liam** lined up his toy cars, but these issues in and of themselves did not result in a definitive diagnosis of ASD. Olivia, Liam, and Noah all underwent evaluations by Early Intervention programs, and were all referred for evaluations for ASD when they were about two and a half to three years old. All three children were tested to have normal hearing and normal vision. During their assessments, additional history, observations of their behavior, and results of the ADOS revealed the following.

Olivia did not use full words, but occasionally used sounds that were similar to words. She was observed to point and gesture to make her needs known. She played with dolls and showed the dolls to the examiner during her play. She responded to directions – for example, "feed the baby." She vocalized animal sounds for toy animals (woof, woof; meow) and had them play with dolls. Olivia was not diagnosed with autism, but instead with a speech-language delay and also sensitivity to some noises/auditory input.

Liam's early learning and communication testing scores were all above average. He did not qualify for early Intervention services. When his parents asked what they should do when he lines up cars, they were encouraged to distract him with other activities so he did not get "stuck" on this activity.

Noah's eye contact was limited. He did not consistently respond to his name. He did not use single words to communicate, though he did sometimes randomly express what professionals call jargoning, making noises like "budabudabuda." He did not point to make his needs known. When he wanted something, he took his mother's forearm and brought her to what he wanted but did not look at his mother or the desired object. When he was given a toy car, he held the toy car very close to the side of his face, looking at it with a sideward glance and focused on spinning the wheels. Instead of placing pieces into a form puzzle board, he flipped the pieces in a repetitive manner. The examiner felt that Noah met criteria for the diagnosis of ASD.

Olivia, Liam, and Noah all had additional evaluations, i.e., "second opinions," regarding their diagnoses.

Olivia was shy with her second examiner. She hid behind her mother and would not separate from her to participate in the assessment. This behavior made it difficult to reach a definitive diagnosis. However, an evaluation provided by the public schools indicated that Olivia's testing scores and survey results fell within normal limits for her age with the significant exception of speech-language testing. These results were consistent with Olivia's initial diagnosis of an expressive language disorder. She did not appear to meet criteria for ASD.

Liam was very interested in many of the toys in the second examiner's room. Although he changed toys frequently, he shared them with the examiner and described his play. Liam did not present with social, language, or behavioral atypicalities, and the examiner did not feel that Liam met criteria for ASD.

At his second evaluation, Noah's examiner agreed that he met criteria for the diagnosis of ASD. Special education and specialized therapies were recommended. In addition, some laboratory testing, including genetic testing, was suggested.

WHAT CAUSES AUTISM SPECTRUM DISORDER?

Trying to establish a single, specific cause for autism is complex – and might not be possible. A positive family history of ASD may be a contributing factor. Having a family member who has been diagnosed with ASD increases the likelihood of ASD in a child. Some specific genetic syndromes also increase the risk for autism. If a child has been diagnosed with ASD, diagnostic testing to assess for specific syndromes and other medical diagnoses is typically completed after a full history and physical exam are completed. Children with other developmental and neurological disorders may also be at risk of presenting with features of autism spectrum disorder. Some genetic syndromes and other medical diagnoses associated with ASD have distinct physical, medical, and genetic features – for example, Fragile X syndrome, mutations in the PTEN gene, Tuberous Sclerosis. Details about these diagnoses are beyond the scope of this chapter. There have also been concerns publicized regarding environmental causes of ASD, including a concern that childhood immunizations might cause or somehow increase the risk that a child will become autistic. To date, scientific studies have found no link between childhood immunizations and autism.

IN ADDITION TO SOCIAL COMMUNICATION PROBLEMS AND REPETITIVE, SOMEWHAT RIGID BEHAVIORS, WHAT OTHER TYPES OF BEHAVIORAL CHALLENGES CAN BE OBSERVED IN CHILDREN WITH ASD?

Please note: None of these behaviors occurring alone make autism a definitive diagnosis.

Aggression

Children with ASD often have difficulty with regulating their behavior and emotions, which can be associated with outbursts/temper tantrums, self-injurious behaviors, and aggression towards others – biting, hitting, or kicking out of frustration or anger.

Anxiety

Children with ASD can become very anxious, stressed, and upset in response to a change in their routine, such as a substitute teacher, a change in a car route, or school vacation week. Children with ASD can focus intensively on a specific topic – for example, the weather: a child may worriedly and repetitively ask, "Is there going to be a tornado?" Children with ASD can demonstrate unacceptable perseverative/repetitive behaviors, which can be anxiety related, such as picking of skin or twirling/pulling of their hair (or a family member's hair).

Developmental Regression

It is estimated that about 25% of children with ASD have a history of a regression in developmental skills (Hyman et al., 2020), specifically communication and social skills. The regression is often reported to occur between 14 months and two years old.

Hyperactivity and Impulsivity, With Difficulty Regulating Behavior

Children with autism can be overly active and may have a limited understanding of potentially dangerous actions – for example, climbing and jumping on furniture, "bolting" in public places.

Irritability and Difficulty Regulating Emotions

Children with ASD can appear more irritable and more easily upset than typical children. This, in combination with poor emotional and behavioral regulation, can be associated with prolonged tantrums/outbursts with difficulty soothing.

Potty/Bowel-Bladder Training challenges

Children with ASD should be expected to be potty trained at an age that is appropriate for their developmental level. In addition to possible cognitive and language difficulties, the behavioral challenges associated with autism can make potty training difficult.

Repetitive Behaviors/Compulsions/Tics

Repetitive behaviors are included in the criteria for ASD. However, it can sometimes be challenging to differentiate stereotypical behaviors (stereotypies) such as hand flapping from compulsive behaviors such as opening and closing doors or motor and vocal tics such as frequent episodes of eye blinking, facial grimacing, or throat clearing. Although tics are not specific to children with ASD, these types of behaviors can also be observed in children with ASD.

Restrictive Diet, With Sensitivities to Texture, Temperature, and/or Color

Children with autism can be restrictive in their intake. For example, they may prefer foods that are white or beige in color or prefer only "crunchy" or only soft foods. If a child's diet becomes too restrictive, their nutritional status can be compromised. Feeding therapy for children with ASD often requires a sensory-behaviorally-based approach – for example, gradually modifying preferred foods or reward and praise for the child initially allowing a nonpreferred food close to their plate, then on their plate, then touching their lips momentarily, etc.

Sleep Problems

Children with ASD are at increased risk for sleep problems, including difficulty falling asleep, difficulty staying asleep, and early morning awakenings. Behavioral interventions, including establishment of a structured bedtime routine and encouraging a child to fall asleep in their own bed can be challenging for typical children and even more challenging for children with ASD. It has been reported that there is benefit from parental implementation of behavioral interventions to address sleep (Malow et al., 2014), but the family stress that can result from a child's sleep challenges should not be understated.

Wandering/Elopement and Running Off/"Bolting"

A decreased understanding of environmental safety, impulsiveness, and sometimes perseverative interests can result in children with ASD being at an increased risk for wandering/elopement, as well as impulsively running off or "bolting." These behaviors pose a safety risk, including an increased risk of traffic-related injuries and drowning. Anderson and colleagues completed an online survey of families of children with ASD, and close to one-half of the children between four and ten years had a history of elopement, with half of those children being missing long enough for the police to be contacted. Reasons for elopement given by parents included pursuit of an intense interest, leaving an undesired event or location, attempting to go to a desired location, and/or enjoyment of running/movement. Elopement is reported to increase with the severity of ASD, as well as presence of an intellectual disability (Anderson et al., 2012).

CHARACTERISTICS OF ASD CAN SOMETIMES BE OBSERVED IN TYPICALLY DEVELOPING CHILDREN AND ALSO CHILDREN WITH OTHER DIAGNOSES

Children may display some behaviors commonly associated with ASD without meeting criteria for the diagnosis. If only one specific behavior occurs but not others, a diagnosis of autism is unlikely. In order to receive a diagnosis of autism, a child should not be exhibiting behaviors consistent with this diagnosis in only one setting.

Some behaviors that are observed in children with an autism diagnosis can and do appear in children who are not autistic. This makes it even more confusing for parents and caregivers. The professional who is performing the evaluation will assess the quality of the behaviors being examined. Are they frequent? What impact do they have on a child's functioning? These kinds of questions are vital in determining if the behaviors being examined represent variations of typical development or indicate autism. Let us look at some of the features of ASD that are sometimes observed in typically developing children and also may be observed in children with other diagnoses.

Differences in Communication and Social Skills

Children with the diagnosis of a social (pragmatic) communication disorder present with communication challenges that overlap with the diagnosis of ASD, but they do not share the behavioral atypicalities (American Psychiatric Association, 2013; Hyman et al., 2020).

Children with an intellectual developmental disorder typically present with delays in multiple areas, including their communication and social skills. In addition, it is reported that 30% of children with ASD are also diagnosed with ID, and that children with ID are often diagnosed at a younger age (Hyman et al., 2020). Presenting with severe developmental delays can sometimes pose a challenge in making a diagnosis of ASD, resulting in over-diagnosing or underdiagnosing ASD.

Even if a child is not presenting with global delays, children who acquire language skills more slowly may have difficulty socializing with their peers. These delays do not definitively indicate an autism diagnosis, particularly if a child demonstrates an intent to communicate by establishing eye contact, pointing, gesturing, and making vocalizations. Sometimes these children may prefer to play alone because it is easier for them than trying to interact with peers if their language skills are immature. Children with ASD typically have limitations in their connection with others, their intent to communicate, and their interest in communicating with words, sounds, or gestures.

Social difficulties can appear in all kinds of children. Childhood shyness may create social awkwardness. Children, including typically developing children, may avoid talking to less familiar peers or adults. They might avoid making eye contact and/or cover their faces. Behavior such as hiding behind a parent when being asked to say hello to an unfamiliar person can often be seen in typically developing children. Children commonly become shy, anxious, and/or unsure about what to say. Such behaviors are different from those exhibited by children with ASD.

Children are learning and practicing social behaviors as they grow and develop. They often watch peers, older children, and adults to learn how to interact with others. They also often "try out" behaviors to see what will happen. For example, young children make silly sounds with their voices or bodies and use silly voices, watching to see how people around them respond. Do others laugh, pay more attention to the child, include the child after this behavior? In other situations, behaviors like these occur when children become uncomfortable or unsure how to act. As their social skills mature, children might not need to "try out" such behaviors because they have learned that making silly sounds or voices is not acceptable in certain settings (for example, in a classroom). Children go through a complex learning process as they develop social skills. Their behaviors sometimes look odd to others but do not necessarily indicate a diagnosis of autism. Children may demonstrate behaviors that are considered inappropriate, unusual, and/or bothersome to others, but may fall within a normal range of development.

Atypical Behaviors

Children with ASD often display repetitive behaviors called stereotypies. A stereotypy, also described as a "self-stimulatory" behavior, is a repetitive movement such as hand flapping or spinning. Typically developing children do sometimes exhibit repetitive types of behaviors. For example, a child may flap his hands when he is excited. That behavior in and of itself does not necessarily mean that a child is autistic. Moreover, repetitive behaviors may also stem from other diagnoses – for example, motor and vocal tics may be transient or suggestive of a tic disorder; obsessive and compulsive behaviors may suggest an alternative mental health diagnosis.

Sensory-Related Issues

Some children may dislike the feeling of tags on clothing or sand stuck to wet feet. They may struggle with having their hair brushed or nails clipped. They may cover their ears or even cry in response to certain noises. Although children with ASD frequently demonstrate sensory sensitivities, these traits can also appear in typically developing children. Similarly, some children seem to seek out strong, intense input through their senses by jumping, rocking, spinning, playing roughly/wrestling, and/or tight pressure such as a forceful hug or teeth grinding – sensations that seem to provide comfort. Some children may have a better understanding about where their bodies are and how to move them when they receive sensory types of input.

While these types of behaviors are often seen in autistic children, they can also appear in typically developing children. What professionals evaluate when considering a possible diagnosis of autism is the frequency and intensity with which these behaviors occur, and whether they fall within the range of typical development. When such behaviors interfere with or interrupt a child's daily activities and functioning, intervention and evaluation becomes warranted.

In all of the above examples, the same behaviors occur in both children with ASD and typically developing children. Whether the behaviors can be considered "normal" or possible autistic traits hinges on the quality of the behaviors in question. Professionals evaluate the intensity, frequency, and consistency with which the behaviors occur. If a child's behaviors do not limit/interfere with the child's everyday functioning, the child will not likely meet criteria for the diagnosis of autism (Morrison, 2014). Some children seem to "march to the beat of a different drummer." However, if you ask the child's teacher how he or she feels the child's social skills, behavior, and ability to communicate are developing compared to their peers, and the response is that there have been no significant concerns, it is not very likely that the child is on the autism spectrum.

In addition to the wide range of behaviors that can be observed in children who are typically developing that may overlap with some features of ASD, other diagnoses can also share features with autism, adding to the complexity of whether a diagnosis of autism may be warranted. Some of these alternative diagnoses include communication disorders, an intellectual disability, ADHD, and posttraumatic stress disorder (PTSD). Children exhibiting certain behaviors may "look" as though they are exhibiting signs of ASD but in fact may be exhibiting features of another diagnosis. For example, a child who displays limited vocal interactions with others may have a communication disorder or an ID. Similarly, a child who fidgets with his/her hands rapidly and repeatedly and cannot seem to sit still may be exhibiting signs of ADHD. A child who is excessively withdrawn, quiet, and avoiding of others may not be autistic, but instead, could be presenting with childhood shyness of even PTSD.

Parents are not expected to diagnose their own children, but they should be aware that some of the "concerning" behaviors they may observe in their child might not indicate ASD, but instead may be considered within the spectrum of "typical" development, or may be indicative of another disorder. As a professional you can help parents differentiate among these possible diagnoses.

It is also important to remember that children with hearing or vision challenges can present with delays in their skills and sometimes appear to present atypically. **It is important for any child who presents with delays in their skills to have their hearing and vision assessed.**

Finally, it appears worth repeating that some children diagnosed with ASD in early childhood, no longer meet criteria for ASD by young adulthood (Hyman et al., 2020). Although it is difficult to sort out whether individuals who "outgrow" the diagnosis may have been originally misdiagnosed, Hyman and colleagues reported that a change in diagnosis is more likely in children who were diagnosed before 30 months or had been previously diagnosed with PDD based on DSM-IV criteria. It was also reported that stronger cognitive and communication skills, participation in early intervention, and a decrease in repetitive behaviors over time tended to be characteristics of individuals who no longer met criteria for ASD.

AUTHORS' COMMENTARY

Instead of the diagnosis of ASD becoming easier to understand over the past 30 years, it has appeared to us that the complexity of the diagnosis has increased. It has not been unusual for us to observe children diagnosed with ASD who would have just been labeled as "quirky" earlier in our careers. This is not being stated in a judgmental or critical manner – for example, after personally diagnosing a child with ASD, we have later stated to caregivers that it is no longer felt that the child meets criteria for the diagnosis, i.e., we no longer agree with our own diagnosis. It is also interesting to note that when this has occurred, the caregiver often requests that the diagnosis not be "taken away," as the child has benefitted from the intensive services they have received based on this diagnosis. Finally, the term "neurodiversity" has become increasingly used in public literature. We support the idea that people think and interact with the world in different ways, and whether or not the differences are a result of a specific diagnosis, they should be respected and understood. Accepting and encouraging individuality can be positive goals, but if an individual's differences are having a negative impact on their functioning, providing supports to improve their quality of life can be beneficial.

ARE CHILDREN WITH ASD AT AN INCREASED RISK FOR MEDICAL PROBLEMS?

In addition to behavioral issues associated with ASD, there have been some medical issues that have been reported to occur more frequently in children with ASD. In 2018, Soke and colleagues reported on the prevalence of medical as well as behavioral symptoms in both four and eight-year-old children with ASD based on 2010 data from five sites of the ADDM Network. In addition to the behavioral issues that are considered known characteristics of the diagnosis and the increased risk for the behavioral and mental health diagnoses discussed above – i.e., language disorder, feeding and sleep challenges; self-injurious behaviors; sensory integration disorder; developmental regression; cognitive/intellectual disability; symptoms of ADHD, oppositional-defiant disorder (ODD), and anxiety; and aggressive behaviors – children with ASD were also reported to be at increased risk for seizures, gastrointestinal problems, and genetic syndromes (Soke et al., 2018). In our experience any central nervous system-based developmental diagnosis, such as ID or ASD, increases a child's risk for other central nervous system-based diagnoses – for example, seizures. Gastrointestinal complaints such as gastro-esophageal reflux and constipation and feeding problems, both restrictive and over-eating, are not uncommonly reported in children with ASD. However, it is notable that in a 2009 population-based study, it was concluded that the data suggested that the etiology of the higher incidence of gastrointestinal symptoms of constipation and food selectivity in children with ASD was more likely to have a neurobehavioral than an organic gastrointestinal etiology (Ibrahim et al., 2009). In another study, Holingue and colleagues examined reports of gastrointestinal problems in children with ASD, comparing those with an ID and those without. Parental reports regarding objective signs such as constipation, diarrhea, and emesis/spitting up were not significantly different between the groups (Holingue et al., 2023).

WHAT TYPES OF SUPPORTS, INTERVENTIONS, AND THERAPIES ARE AVAILABLE FOR CHILDREN WITH AUTISM SPECTRUM DISORDER?

There is no "cure" for autism. Scientific articles and popular press have featured various treatments and interventions. Several categories of treatment intervention have become available, including educational interventions, behavioral interventions, medication, and alternative treatments. Some parents rely exclusively on one or another type of intervention, but more frequently, caregivers use a combination of interventions to support their child who has been diagnosed with ASD.

BEHAVIORAL THERAPIES/TECHNIQUES AND EDUCATIONAL PROGRAMS

Multiple interventions have been endorsed to treat children with ASD, some of which have been studied and are considered evidence-based. Children who have been diagnosed with ASD before the age of three will qualify for early intervention services, and those diagnosed after the age of three will be provided with an individualized education program (IEP) for preschool. Specific services will be determined by the type and severity of a child's needs. A range of educational techniques, therapies, and supports have emerged to help children with ASD and their families. It is important that families work with early intervention and/or schoolteachers and therapists to explore the available therapies and programs in order to decide which is the most optimal for their children. Treatments and therapies are sometimes categorized as Comprehensive or Direct (Hyman et al., 2020); some are classroom-based, some are natural environment-based; some have been studied more scientifically and are considered evidenced-based. The following are some ASD treatments, programs, and therapies, some designed specifically for children with ASD and some as possibly adjunct therapies. They have been listed alphabetically.

Applied Behavior Analysis (ABA) Therapy

This is an intensive therapy that involves systematically and repetitively applying interventions and reinforcement in order to decrease specific unacceptable behaviors and improve acceptable ones. ABA implements positive reinforcement to create positive behavioral changes. This therapy has been studied and has been considered the evidence-based/standard therapy for children with ASD. There is evidence that early and intensive ABA intervention can improve outcomes for children with ASD, including improvements in socialization and communication skills (Yu et al., 2020). However, despite the reported benefits, ABA has also recently been the target of some concerns. We therefore feel that it is important to spend time discussing this particular therapy in more detail.

Ole Ivar Lovaas, a Norwegian American clinical psychologist who worked with children with autism in the 1960s, is known for first introducing some of the origins of ABA therapy. However, some of the children treated by Lovaas received punishments/aversive treatments, including electric shocks. In 1987 Lovaas used discrete trial training (DTT) to treat what were reported to be unacceptable behaviors demonstrated by individuals with autism (Lovaas, 1987; Winter, 2024). Discrete trial training involves breaking down a skill into smaller elements/units and then using a series of direct, systematic instructions repeatedly until a skill is acquired. Discrete trial training laid the foundation for ABA therapy.

Over the past 30 to 40 years, there have been multiple reports advocating the benefits of ABA therapy for children with ASD (Lotfizadeh et al., 2018; Yu et al., 2020). This has included anecdotal reports as well as evidence-based information from retrospective and randomized control studies. Children with ASD who were provided with ABA therapy in randomized controlled trials benefitted from the therapy, and studies indicated children with ASD were found to be more likely to achieve the goals identified by their programs. It was also reported that improvements were related to receiving ABA therapy for multiple hours pers week, from 15 hours to sometimes as many as 40 hours per week, for an extended period of time, generally 12 to 24 months (Linstead et al., 2017; Orinstein et al., 2014; Ospina et al., 2008; Yu et al., 2020). In 2020, Yu and colleagues completed a meta-analysis of 14 randomized controlled trials of several therapies that incorporate the principles of ABA therapy. The results suggested outcomes of socialization, communication, and expressive language may be "promising targets" for ABA-based interventions involving children with ASD (significant improvements in other areas were not reported) (Yu et al., 2020). It is notable that the techniques of ABA therapy have been incorporated into several other therapies, some of which were included in Yu's analysis. Retrospective studies have also supported intensive ABA services.

As a result of an increasing amount of literature about ASD in the public, the ASD diagnosis becoming more common, published evidence of ABA therapy, as well as the support of parent and advocacy groups, more support for individuals with autism has been provided over the past 15 to 20 years, and this has included improved access to ABA therapy and educational programs. Public laws have included the Combating Autism Act of 2006 (Public Law 109–416) and its reauthorization in 2011, authorizing funds for services and research for individuals with ASD. In 2014 The Autism Collaboration, Accountability, Research, Education and Support (CARES) Act reauthorized the Combating Autism act, which allocated funds for research dedicated to the diagnosis of ASD and training in evidence-based practices for individuals with ASD (Public Law 113–157); the law was reauthorized in 2019 (Public Law 116–60). The majority of states developed licensure for certified behavior analysts to treat children with ASD (Hyman et al., 2020). Professionals who are specifically certified in behavioral analysis typically create individualized ABA programs for children with ASD and also supervise the individuals who provide the therapy. State mandates were gradually created, with the goal of expanding insurance coverage for ASD services including ABA therapy (Barry et al., 2017; Choi et al., 2020). As of 2022, all 50 states in the U.S. implemented Medicaid insurance coverage for treatment of individuals with ASD, with most states covering ABA therapy. Although state mandates include coverage of services by commercial insurance companies, some commercial insurances are exempt from covering this service. Variability in coverage of ABA among states and insurance plans remains.

Despite the positive anecdotal and evidence-based reports regarding the benefits of ABA, there have also been concerns reported. Even with state mandates, the amount of ABA therapy that children are able to receive is variable. There are insurance coverage exemptions, sometimes long waiting lists for therapy, a shortage of available certified therapists, and inconsistent coverage among commercial insurers. It has also been noted that data based on randomized-controlled studies may have challenges in their applicability to clinical settings. Choi and colleagues (2020) retrospectively examined data regarding ABA services in California, a state where there is mandated commercial insurance coverage. They identified "real world" challenges to implementing ABA: 13% of referred children received no ABA, two-thirds of children who received ABA continued services for 12 months, and less than half continued services for 24 months. In addition, the children often received a relatively lower than recommended number of hours of therapy per week. Of note, however, despite the limitation in services, the children with the lowest adaptive level at baseline made clinically and statistically significant gains in their skills. The reason for discontinuation of services was not typically a result of poor progress; it was reported that having a parent who was married/partnered increased the odds of remaining in ABA for 12 and 24 months, suggesting that caregiver support may play a role in service continuation.

In addition to the challenges accessing ABA therapy, there have also been concerns reported regarding the therapy itself. Lovaas' original aversive techniques (as well as reported negative descriptions of his patients) are considered unacceptable. But even the more modern error ABA techniques have been criticized by some individuals with ASD and their families, sometimes as a part of the current "neurodiversity movement." The therapy has been reported by some to be a negative experience as the therapy requires long hours of repetitive tasks and may teach participants that some of an individual with ASD's unique or "quirky" behaviors are unacceptable and require change to become more "acceptable behaviors" (Winter, 2024).

It is notable that there are also additional specific interventions and programs designed for children with ASD that incorporate ABA techniques, some of which will be discussed later in this section.

AUTHORS' COMMENTARY

In our experience there are still challenges to accessing ABA therapy, particularly regarding long waiting lists and insurance coverage. In our clinical experience, children with more severe symptoms of ASD, such as self-injurious behaviors, aggression, and bolting, often appear to benefit greatly from the intensive therapeutic techniques included in ABA. The efficacy of the therapy for children whose features of ASD include mostly communication and social challenges in combination with some stereotypies and specific interests appear less certain. We have also observed that ABA techniques may also be beneficial for some children without ASD – for example, poorly regulated children who demonstrate aggressive, acting out behaviors. However, ABA therapy is typically only available for children who have a definitive diagnosis of ASD.

Cognitive Behavioral Therapy (CBT)

This is an evidence-based therapy that devises strategies to address specific behaviors needing alteration. This is not a therapy designed specifically for children with ASD, but can sometimes be useful as part of their treatment program. This approach begins by identifying specific problem behaviors. Therapy focuses on reducing problem behaviors and/or thoughts, while at the same time increasing positive behaviors and thought patterns. Efforts to decrease problematic behaviors are made by implementing desensitization strategies and strengthening coping strategies and problem-solving skills. Relaxation and visualization strategies are often included in this type of therapy. Cognitive behavioral therapy is most often implemented to address anxiety and may not be as effective or appropriate for some individuals with more severe intellectual disabilities.

Developmental Relationship-Focused Interventions

These interventions focus on a caregiver's responsiveness as it relates to a child's development of social communication. This developmental model promotes social development through coaching to increase a child's responsiveness to an adult using activities such as imitation and play (Landry et al., 2000; Siller & Sigman. 2002; Tamis-LeMonda et al., 2001). The models emphasize social reciprocity (Solomon et al., 2014). Some of the developmental relationship-based approaches used for children with ASD include Developmental, Individual-differences, Relationship-based/Floortime

(DIR/Floortime), Relationship Development Intervention (RDI), and the Social Communication/Emotional Regulation/Transactional Supports model (SCERTS).

Developmental, Individual-Differences, Relationship-Based/Floortime (DIR/Floortime)

Sometimes referred to as **Floortime**, this is a relationship-based therapy that has been implemented for children with ASD. The intervention utilizes play and social engagement in attempts to improve human connections and facilitate social-emotional and developmental skills – for example, self-regulation, communication, and reasoning. Floortime can be done in a child's natural environment. Solomon and colleagues completed a randomized controlled trial comparing parenting coaching using the techniques of DIR/Floortime with controls in children aged between two and five. Parents who were taught this approach were less directive, and their children were rated as more socially responsive; there was no difference in IQ and language scores between groups, and half of the children in the control group also improved in their affective ratings (Hyman et al., 2020; Solomon, et al., 2014).

Relationship Development Intervention (RDI)

This is a family-based behavioral treatment, developed by Dr. Steven Gutstein, that focuses on building the social and emotional skills of children with ASD (Gutstein, 2009).

Social Communication/Emotional Regulation/ Transactional Support (SCERTS)

This is an educational model developed by Barry Prizant, PhD, Amy Wetherby, PhD, Emily Rubin, and Amy Laurant. SCERTS utilizes principles from other teaching models (including ABA and Treatment and Education of Autistic and related Communication-Handicapped Children [TEACCH]) and promotes child-initiated communication in daily activities (Prizant et al., 2006).

Early Start Denver Model (ESDM)

This intervention incorporates the principles of infant and toddler development into play and daily routines. ESDM is considered a **Naturalistic Developmental Behavioral Intervention (NDBI)** that incorporates some ABA techniques to facilitate developmentally based learning and social skills. The intervention is provided in a child's natural environments and uses child-initiated teaching opportunities (Schreibman et al., 2015). The techniques of this model facilitate developmental skills during daily activities and play, while decreasing the symptoms of ASD that often negatively impact a child's ability to learn, communicate, and make social connections. The strategies incorporate interpersonal exchanges using natural materials and activities. Adults are sensitive to, and respond to, the child's verbal and nonverbal cues, and the model addresses all developmental areas. ESDM intervention techniques can be implemented by both therapists and parents. The intervention integrates play and a relationship approach with the principles of ABA therapy and is individualized based on a child's developmental profile (Rogers & Dawson, 2010). In a multisite trial of ESDM, early age and more hours of total therapy were associated with improved outcome (Rogers et al., 2012).

Functional Behavioral Assessment/Analysis (FBA)

This is an observational assessment that is often the first step in addressing specific behavioral problems. This assessment is not designed specifically for children with ASD but can be useful to create a behavioral plan for a child who is demonstrating one or more negative behaviors. This analysis is typically completed by a behavioral specialist at school. The observation explores the events and conditions that typically precede specific behaviors, i.e., possible precipitants/causes, and what happens as a result of the behavior (for example, the child receives attention, avoids a nonpreferred activity, etc.). A plan based on the observations is then created with interventions designed to decrease the maladaptive/negative behaviors. For example, an FBA might indicate that a child is hitting their own head to gain attention from the caregiver. A plan could then be designed in which the child receives direct attention when doing an appropriate activity for a brief period of time. This plan would give the child the opportunity to get what they want (attention) while doing what the caregiver wants (appropriate behavior). The goal is to teach the child over time that doing an appropriate behavior or activity will get them the desired reward/attention (Fox & Gable, 2004). Completion of an FBA is not specific to children with ASD – this type of analysis can be completed to address negative behaviors in children with and without specific diagnoses.

Learning Experiences and Alternate Program for Preschoolers and their Parents (LEAP) Model

This is an inclusive educational program where typically developing children are taught to facilitate the social skills and communication of children with ASD. LEAP blends principles of ABA with special and general education teaching techniques for pupils in inclusive settings (Boyd et al., 2014; Strain & Bovey, 2011). Family members are also taught these techniques, which can include Picture Exchange Communication System (PECS), Pivotal Response Training, incidental teaching, and peer mediated interventions. A randomized controlled trial of preschool-aged children revealed that LEAP was associated with improvement in socialization, cognition, language, and challenging behaviors compared to standard methods (teachers were given only a LEAP manual) (Strain & Bovey, 2011).

Parent Management Training

Parent management training can take the form of providing parental supports, as well as **parent mediated interventions**. **Parent support interventions** include care coordination and education, while **parent mediated training** involves teaching parents and other caregivers interventions as part of a child's therapeutic program. Interventions may involve ABA techniques in a child's natural environment (Bearss et al., 2015a). There have been several randomized controlled trials for these types of therapies (Beaudoin et al., 2014; Bearss et al., 2015a; Bearss et al., 2015b; Oono et al., 2013; Smith & Iadarola, 2015). Results of a randomized controlled trial of toddlers and their caregivers revealed that hands on parent training in the concepts of joint attention, child engagement and regulation, and symbolic play with their child for 10 weeks was superior to a parent-only psychoeducational intervention in the area of joint attention (Kasari et al., 2015). A parent training approach can assist in improving program goals and may be used to promote improvements in child and caregiver goals (Bearss et al., 2013; Bearss et al., 2015a; Grahame et al., 2015; Harrop, 2015; Scahill et al., 2016).

Picture Exchange Communication System (PECS)

This is an exchange-based communication system that is often used for children with limited language skills, including children with ASD. Children are provided with pictures and are taught to give the picture to another person in exchange for the desired item, encouraging and facilitating a child's ability to initiate communication. This system also incorporates some ABA-based techniques (Flippin et al., 2010; Hyman et al., 2020).

Pivotal Response Treatment (PRT)

This is an intervention that uses a child's natural motivators – for example, toys, games, preferred activities – to teach and reinforce new, socially appropriate behaviors. The treatment incorporates the principles of ABA, but is play-based and uses natural rewards/reinforcements. It focuses on "pivotal" points/moments in a child's development in order to make changes in a child's behavior (Verschuur et al., 2014).

Sensory Integration Therapy

This grew out of the work of A. Jean Ayres, PhD, OTR. This type of therapy helps children gather and process sensory information from their environment (i.e., sights, sounds, smells, touch, taste) as well as movement, and respond to it in an appropriate way. It can be particularly beneficial for children who are over-responsive or under-responsive to sensory input (Ayres & Robbins, 1979).

Social Stories

This technique was first devised by Carol Gray in 1991. A Social Story is a social learning tool for exchanging information about a personalized topic. It is written by a caregiver in a way that is safe and meaningful for a child with ASD. Social Stories are typically written about a topic that is relevant to the individual child. The specific topic may be particularly stressful and/or difficult for the child, and can be addressed through a story that is meant to be comforting and informative. The intent is to provide honest information to children in a way that provides understanding and makes them feel physically, socially, and emotionally safe (Gray & Garand, 1993).

Social Skills Instruction

Deficits in social skills and social communication are included in the criteria for ASD (American Psychiatric Association, 2013; Morrison, 2014). Teaching social skills has therefore become a part of programs for many children with ASD. Social skills can be taught individually and/or as part of a group, and instruction can be at home, at school, as part of counseling, or within other community resources. Teaching social skills can be part of therapies and interventions provided by counselors, social workers, psychologists, speech-language pathologists, teachers, and caregivers. Improving a child's social skills is often included as one of the goals for children with ASD. It can be included in a child's IEP or 504 Accommodation Plan and can also be provided in settings outside of school. Interventions may include adult-mediated or peer-mediated social skill building, or a combination of both. Child-directed social skills interventions are often delivered individually or in small groups with other children with similar needs (Foster & Pearson, 2012; Kasari et al., 2012; Kretzmann et al., 2015; Otero et al., 2015; Reichow et al., 2013; Whalon et al., 2015). Goals of therapy may include improving a child's ability to recognize social cues, teaching strategies for social problem-solving, and implementing cognitive-behavioral techniques (Otero et al., 2015). Results of a randomized controlled study reported in 2012 revealed an improvement in social skills in children with and without ASD who were provided with social skills training in natural social group environments such as in the classroom or on the playground (Kasari et al., 2012). The Program for the Education and Enrichment of Relational Skills is an evidence-based group approach in teaching social skills that has been reported to have some impact on improving social functioning of adolescents (Laugeson et al., 2014). Reichow and colleagues completed a systematic review of randomized controlled trials of social skills training for children aged 6 to 21 years, and results revealed that interventions improved social competence and friendship quality but did not result in differences in emotional recognition and social communication. In addition, the transfer of skills to other settings was inconsistent (Reichow et al., 2013).

Speech-Language Therapy

This is an essential component of educational programs for any child with a speech-language delay or disorder. Since communication challenges are included in the criteria for ASD, speech-language therapy should always be a part of a child's treatment program. In addition to verbal language, this approach teaches the use of nonverbal communication techniques, including using pictures, signs, gestures, and augmentative communication devices, to facilitate communication for children who have limited or no verbal communication skills. For example, by using communication applications on electronic devices, children learn to make their choices and desires known by pushing buttons. Using their hands to form a sign might allow nonverbal children to communicate that they are finished with an activity or that they want more to eat.

Treatment and Education of Autistic and Related Communication-Handicapped Children (TEACCH)

This was developed by Eric Schopler and colleagues at the University of North Carolina at Chapel Hill in the early 1970s. TEACCH is an educational method based on the observation that children with ASD tend to be visual learners. Structured teaching in this program provides students with an understanding of their environment, a specific schedule, and behavior-based instruction (Mesibov et al., 2004). Classroom settings are visually organized in order to promote engagement of students (Boyd et al., 2014). By organizing the environment and providing a predictable schedule, the program attempts to minimize distractions, improve regulation, decrease frustration, facilitate learning, and promote independence (Boyd et al. 2014; Strain & Hoyson, 2000; Strain & Bovey, 2011; Virues-Ortego et al., 2013). This approach has been associated with some benefit for students with ASD in their perceptual, motor, verbal, and cognitive skills, with less effect reported in adaptive and motor function and challenging behaviors (Virues-Ortega et al., 2013).

A comparison of the effects of LEAP and TEACCH classrooms with those of standard special education classes taught by teachers familiar with ASD revealed that the common features of these interventions may be responsible for improvements observed in all students. TEACCH was associated with more reported improvement of ASD features for students who had greater intellectual deficits (Boyd et al., 2014).

Final note: Although there are some educational and therapy programs that strictly implement one specific treatment, many programs use a combined approach – for example, principles of ABA combined with speech-language therapy, PECS, participation in a social skills group, and parent training in order to meet the individual needs of a child with ASD.

MEDICATIONS

No single medication "treats" or "cures" autism, but various medications do treat specific associated behavioral challenges. Caution should be used when treating children with medication, as each medication can potentially be associated with negative side effects.

Psychostimulant medications, such as methylphenidate and dextroamphetamine, can both decrease a child's activity level and impulsivity as well as improve a child's ability to focus and pay attention. Atypical antipsychotics medications have been studied in children with autism. Risperidone has been approved for treatment of severe behavioral dysregulation in children with autism, but individuals need to be monitored closely for potential negative side effects. Some kinds of alpha-adrenergic medications, such as extended release/long acting guanfacine, can sometimes be beneficial in treating hyperactivity and impulsivity. It is notable that results of a recent meta-analysis of interventions targeting irritability in children with various mental health diagnoses, including ASD, ADHD, disruptive behavior disorders, disruptive mood dysregulation disorder, and severe mood dysregulation, revealed that the largest effects were shown for children with ASD (Breaux et al., 2023).

ALTERNATIVE THERAPIES

Additional therapies that may be offered for a child who has been diagnosed with ASD include hippotherapy (therapeutic horseback riding), aqua therapy, music therapy, art therapy, pet/animal therapy, and other recreation-based therapies. Supplemental therapies such as therapeutic horseback riding and swimming are often beneficial for children with developmental challenges, including children with ASD. Although all of these alternative therapies may not be evidence-based, they can be fun and engaging for children, providing opportunities for relaxation, improved coordination, and social interactions.

Diet and Dietary Supplements

Some sources in the media and parent networks have endorsed dietary modifications and non-medication supplements as having possible benefits for children with autism. Parents should be advised to **proceed with caution** when considering dietary or non-medication treatments that:

- are offered as a "cure" for autism, particularly if the treatment is also described as curing multiple unrelated diagnoses;
- include a very restrictive dietary regimen, particularly for a child who is already restrictive in his intake (the diet may increase the child's risk of suboptimal nutrition – for example, the nutrition of a child who only eats white or beige foods and liquids may be at risk of being suboptimal if he is placed on a casein- and gluten-free diet);
- require families to pay large sums of money for certain diets (families may be taken advantage of in their quest to help their child).

CASE STUDIES

At 3 years old, **Olivia** qualified for participation in an inclusion preschool program with an IEP based on her delays in communication. She received speech-language therapy twice a week as part of her school program, once a week individually and once a week in a small group. She demonstrated improvements in all of her skills. By the time Olivia started kindergarten, her language was age-appropriate and she no longer qualified for an IEP.

Liam continued to sometimes line up his cars, but he also engaged in other activities. He did well in preschool. Although he was considered a high achiever and somewhat "perfectionistic," there were no concerns regarding his social, behavioral, or learning status throughout his schooling.

At three years old, **Noah** was enrolled in a full-day special education preschool program that included speech-language therapy, occupational therapy, and ABA therapy. After school he also received in-home ABA therapy four days a week. Noah demonstrated improvements in all of his skills.

ADVICE FOR PARENTS

When a parent is considering trying a particular therapy, advise them to ask their child's pediatrician about any scientific information that may be available.

Other parents can be very helpful when exploring supports for a child. However, parents should keep in mind that when other parents have spent time and finances on a specific therapy, they can sometimes lose objectivity about its benefits.

"HELPFUL HINTS" FOR TEACHERS AND PRACTITIONERS

If a child's parents are endorsing features of autism but you do not observe behaviors that make the diagnosis definitive you should:

- obtain information from other professionals who are currently working with or have previously worked with the child;
- keep in mind that there are other diagnoses with features that overlap with autism;

- ask a parent to videotape some of the concerning behaviors they are observing at home;
- explore services available for children with alternative diagnoses and behavioral problems (if the parents are seeking the diagnosis in order for their child to be eligible for services and supports);
- discuss referring the child to an Autism Center for an evaluation.

If you think that a child is presenting with features of autism but the child's parent does not agree:

- review the criteria for the diagnosis;
- explain that features of the diagnosis may change and that therefore a definitive diagnosis does not necessarily need to be made immediately;
- explain that ABA and other programs and therapies may be beneficial for the child, and re-evaluation for this diagnosis will therefore continue over time;
- with parents' permission, request information from professionals who have previously worked with, or are currently working with, the child;
- discuss referring the child to an Autism Center for an evaluation;
- For a child with multiple behavioral issues, work with the parents to prioritize which specific behaviors are most maladaptive and initially focus on those.

Depending on the child's presentation during their assessments, sometimes professionals do not agree on a specific diagnosis. It is important to remember that behavioral and educational interventions can sometimes be determined based on the child's areas of weaknesses regardless of the specific diagnosis.

AUTHORS' COMMENTARY

There are multiple benefits of collaborating with disciplines outside your own profession. With parental permission, ongoing communication with a child's teacher, school therapists, and the school counselor is extremely important in helping a child and their family. By exchanging information regarding each person's observations of a child, the diagnosis of ASD may be able to be confirmed and/or other diagnoses can be considered.

HANDOUT FOR CAREGIVERS

Autism Spectrum Disorder (ASD)

Children with ASD present with weaknesses in social communication and social interaction, together with behaviors that are considered "atypical," including repetitive behaviors and/or movements, inflexibility regarding routines, intense interests in specific subjects/activities, sensory sensitivities, and/or sensory seeking behaviors. The range and number of children who meet criteria for ASD has increased over time, and children can present with mild to more severe symptoms.

Evaluation

Your child's primary care physician may be the first consultant with whom you discuss this diagnosis. The physician may request that you complete questionnaires and they will also complete an initial assessment of your child's behavior and skills. If your child is less than three years old, a referral to early intervention (EI) can be completed. If there are concerns regarding the diagnosis of ASD, a referral for an evaluation specifically for this diagnosis by a psychologist, neuropsychologist, neurologist, developmental-behavioral pediatrician, or neurologist will be completed.

Because there is no specific medical test to confirm a diagnosis of ASD, the road to obtain a diagnosis may not be straightforward. Even when your child has been given a diagnosis of ASD, the journey can be complex, sometimes confusing, but also rewarding.

Common Questions

Is my child's behavior inappropriate, or do I just have limited tolerance?
If a child presents with behavioral problems at home, parents should consider the feedback they have received from their child's teachers or daycare workers – this is true whether or not the child has been diagnosed with ASD. If a child has no reported significant behavior problems at school, this is reassuring. However, if his behavior at home appears problematic, this could be related to the child's increased comfort level at home; it is also possible that parental expectations could be a contributing factor. If a child's behavior has been problematic at home, seeking a professional consultation with a behavioral counselor can help explore which behaviors demonstrated by the child would be appropriate to address.

Will treatment with medication help to alleviate some of my child's behavioral problems?

It is important to determine the degree to which a child's behavior negatively impacts their functioning in all settings. If the child attends a school with appropriate supports and is working with specialists at school and/or outside of school, and multiple individuals have reported that the child's behavior is negatively impacting on their ability to function, a discussion regarding treatment with medication may be appropriate. However, risks need to be reviewed thoroughly with the child's physician.

Can my child be cured or outgrow the diagnosis of ASD?

Although ASD is typically a diagnosis that is not "cured," the presentation of autism may change over time. Sometimes a child who meets criteria for autism at a young age may no longer meet criteria for the diagnosis at a later age. The following are some examples of children who were initially diagnosed with ASD but were no longer felt to meet criteria during later childhood.

- The child presented with a language delay/disorder at a young age, and as their language improved, the behavioral differences resolved.
- The behaviors of a child initially appeared to be characteristics of ASD, including behavioral dysregulation; however, the behaviors were later felt to be more consistent with another developmental or mental health diagnoses – for example, attention-deficit/hyperactivity disorder (ADHD), ADHD in combination with a history of a language disorder, obsessive-compulsive disorder, oppositional defiant disorder, or anxiety disorder.

Why have I received different opinions regarding the diagnosis of ASD?

Autism is a clinical diagnosis. A professional will base their opinion on the child's reported behavior in school and at home, as well as the child's behavior during their visit(s). A child's behavior can be variable and can change with age, therefore a child may appear to meet full criteria for the diagnosis of autism during one assessment, but not during a later assessment, as their communication and behavioral skills may appear different.

My child repeats everything I say – is that "echolalia," a symptom of autism?

Repeating words is a normal way for a child to learn language. Echolalia refers to imitating words in a repetitive manner without communicative intent, without looking at the other individual, and repeating the words in a self-stimulatory, non-functional manner. "Delayed echolalia" involves repeating words and phrases at a later time, again in a repetitive manner without communicative intent. "Scripted language" is the repeating of phrases, sentences, and sometimes longer dialogue that the individual has heard in movies, TV shows, etc. with the "scripting" often not relevant to the situation.

Why has the number of children with ASD increased?

According to research studies, the number of children diagnosed with autism has increased over time. Although one specific cause of the increase is not completely clear, there are many possible contributing factors,

- The definition has changed, and when you change the definition or criteria of a diagnosis, the prevalence of the diagnosis is likely to change. For example, the diagnoses of pervasive developmental disorder (PDD) and Asperger disorder were taken out of the DSM. Most of these children are now considered to have autism spectrum disorder.
- As information about the diagnosis has become more widespread, the diagnosis is considered more frequently than in the past – for example, what was previously considered to be a "quirky personality" in combination with language delays and behavioral concerns, may in more recent years be considered as possibly within the spectrum of autism.
- Professionals may sometimes have a lower threshold for giving a preliminary diagnosis of autism spectrum if they feel that services offered only to children who have been diagnosed with autism spectrum disorder would benefit the child.
- Today's parents are often more aware of the diagnosis, and some parents can have a lower threshold for suspecting this diagnosis. Some parents obtain many assessments in order to confirm that their child's difficulties may be explained by the diagnosis of autism. In addition, in our experience, some parents have commented that it is "easier" to explain a child's issues to other adults by relating that they have been diagnosed with ASD. Because of the media attention that the diagnosis of autism has received in recent years, parents can sometimes feel that the diagnosis of ASD is more comfortable for them than other diagnoses.

My child has an interest in his peers and he wants to make friends. Does that mean he is not on the autism spectrum?

In our experience, it is not unusual for some children with autism spectrum disorder to have a desire to make friends. However, their difficulties in understanding social norms or correctly interpreting language and facial expressions can sometime make this challenging for them. Their differences from peers may result in them not being sought out by their peers. However, with supports, many children on the autism spectrum establish friendships.

I'm concerned that if my child is not diagnosed with autism, he will not be provided with an IEP. What should I do?

Because grassroots and governmental support for children with autism increased, a child who had been diagnosed with ASD may be offered intensive educational and behavioral supports. If a child's IQ and achievement test scores do not qualify the child for an IEP, being diagnosed definitively with ASD may allow the student to qualify; however, this can depend on whether the child's features of ASD are negatively impacting on their school performance and experience. If your child does not qualify for an individualized education program (IEP), there may be other supports available (for example, social skills groups).

My child with ASD has a high intelligence quotient (IQ) and testing results revealed that he is "gifted" in certain areas. Can he still be provided with an IEP?

The diagnosis of ASD can include individuals with above average intelligence, even some who have testing scores in the gifted range. However, the diagnosis includes a weakness in social communication and behavioral challenges that can interfere with a child's ability to function optimally in school. These challenges often require supports in school and, depending on the severity, may qualify a child for an IEP or 504 Accommodation Plan.

Can immunizations cause autism?

Peer-reviewed studies have not supported a link between childhood immunizations and autism.

Note to caregivers: Accepting a child's individuality, while also assisting them and guiding them as they develop into a productive member of society who is able to take advantage of all the positive experiences the world has to offer, can be powerful and rewarding.

BIBLIOGRAPHY

American Psychiatric Association (APA) (2013). *Diagnostic and Statistical Manual of Mental Disorders* – 5th edition. Arlington, VA: American Psychiatric Association Publishing.

American Psychiatric Association (APA) (2022). *Diagnostic and Statistical Manual of Mental Disorders* – *5th edition. Text Revision.* Arlington, VA: American Psychiatric Association Publishing.

Anderson, C., Law, J. K., Daniels, A., Rice, C., Mendell, D. S., Hagopian, L., & Law, P. A. (2012). Occurrence and family impact of elopement in children with autism spectrum disorders. *Pediatrics*, 130(5): 870–877. https://doi.org/10.1542/peds.2012-0762. Epub 2012 Oct 8.

Autism Collaboration, Accountability, Research, Education and Support (CARES) (2014). Public Law 113–157.

Autism Speaks. www.autismspeaks.org.

Autism Society. www.autism-society.org.

Autism Source, Autism Society of America (ASA).

Autism NOW. https://autismnow.org.

Ayres, A. J., & Robbins, J. (1979). *Sensory Integration and the Child*. Los Angeles, Calif: Western Psychological Services.

Barbaresi, W., Cacia, J., Friedman, S., Fussell, J., Hansen, R., Hofer, J., Roizen, N., Stein, R. E. K., Vanderbilt, D., & Sideridis, G. (2022). Clinician diagnostic certainty and the role of the Autism Diagnostic Observation Schedule in autism spectrum disorder diagnosis in young children. *Journal of the American Medical Association (JAMA) Pediatrics*, 176(12): 1233–1241. doi:10.1001/jamapediatrics.2022.3605.

Barry, C. L., Soper, F., Soper, J., Epstein, A. J., Marcus, S. C., Kennedy-Hendricks, A., Candon, M. K., Xie, M., & Mandell, D. S. (2017). Effects of state insurance mandates on health care use and spending for autism spectrum disorder. *Health Affairs (Millwood)*, 36(10): 1754–1761. https://doi.org/10.1377/hlthaff.2017.0515.

Bearss, K., Lecavalier, L., Minshawi, N., Smith, T., Handen, B., Sukhodolsky, D., Aman, M., Swiezy, N., Butter, E., & Scahill, L. (2013). Toward an exportable parent training program for disruptive behaviors in autism spectrum disorders. *Neuropsychiatry (London)*, 3(2): 169–180. doi: 10.2217/npy.13.14.

Bearss, K., Johnson, C., Smith, T., Lecavalier, L., Swiezy, N., Aman, A., McAdam, D. B., Butter, E., Stillitano, C., Minshawi, N., Sukhodolshy, D. G., Mruzek, D.S., Turner, K., Neal, T., Hallett, V., Mulick, J. A., Green, B., Handen, B., Deng, Y. Dziura, J., & Scahill, L. (2015a). Effect of parent training vs parent education on behavioral problems in children with autism spectrum disorder: A randomized clinical trial. *Journal of the American Medical Association*, 313(15): 1524–1533. https://doi.org/10.1001/jama.2015.3150.

Bearss, K., Burrell, T. L., Stewart, L., & Scahill, L. (2015b). Parent training in autism spectrum disorder: What's in a name? *Clinical Child and Family Psychology Review*, 18(2): 170–182. doi: 10.1007/s10567-015-0183-9.

Beaudoin, A. J., Sébire, G., & Couture, M. (2014). Parent training interventions for toddlers with autism spectrum disorder. *Autism Research and Treatment*, 839890.

Boyd, B. A., Hume, K., McBee, M. T., Alessandri, M., Gutierrez, A., Johnson, L., Sperry, L., & Odom, S. L. (2014). Comparative efficacy of LEAP, TEACCH and non-model-specific special education programs for preschoolers with autism spectrum disorders. *Journal of Autism and Developmental Disorders*, 44(2): 366–380. doi: 10.1007/s10803-013-1877-9.

Bradstreet, L. E., Juechter, J. I., Kamphaus, R.W., Kerns, C. M., & Robins, D. L. (2017). Using the BASC-2 parent rating scales to screen for autism spectrum disorder in toddlers and preschool-aged children *Journal of Abnormal Child Psychology*, 45(2): 359–370. doi: 10.1007/s10802-016-0167-3.

Breaux, R., Baweja, R., Hana-May, E., Shroff, D. M., Cash, A. R., Swanson, C. S., Knehans, A., & Waxmonsky, J. G. (2023). Systematic review and meta-analysis: Pharmacological and nonpharmacological interventions for persistent nonepisodic irritability. *Journal of the American Academy of Child and Adolescent Psychiatry*, 62(3): 318–334. doi: 10.1016j.jaac.2022.05.012. Epub 2022 Jun 14.

Bridgemohan, C., Kaufman, B., Johnson, D. M., Shulman, L. H., & Zuckerman, K. E. (2019). *Caring for Children With Autism Spectrum Disorders: A Practical Resource Toolkit for Clinicians – 3rd edition*. Elk Grove, IL: American Academy of Pediatrics.

Choi, K. R., Knight, E. A., Stein, B. D., & Coleman, K. J. (2020). Autism insurance mandates in the US: Comparison of mandated commercial insurance benefits across states. *Maternal and Child Health Journal*, 24(7): 894–900. doi: 10.1007/s10995-020-02950-2. PMID:32356129.

Choi, K. R., Bhakta, B., Knight, E. A., Becerra-Culqui, T. A., Gahre, T. L., Zima, B., & Coleman, K. J. (2022) Patient outcomes after applied behavior analysis for autism spectrum disorder. *Journal of Developmental & Behavioral Pediatrics*, 42(1): 9–16. https://doi.org/10.1097/DBP.0000000000000995.

Combating Autism Act (2006). Public Law 109–416.

Constantino, J. N., Davis, S. A., Todd, R. D., Schindler, M. K., Gross, M. M., Brophy, S. L., Metzger, L. M., Shoushtari, C. S., Splinter, R., & Reich, W. (2003). Validation of a brief quantitative measure of autistic traits: Comparison of the social responsiveness scale with the autism diagnostic interview-revised. *Journal of Autism and Developmental Disorders*, 33(4): 427–433. doi: 10.1023/a:1025014929212.

Corsello, C., Hus, V., Pickles, A., Risi, S., Cook, E. H., Leventhal, B. L., & Lord, C. (2007). Between a ROC and a hard place: Decision making and making decisions about using the SCQ. *Journal of Child Psychology and Psychiatry*, 48(9): 932–940. doi: 10.1111/j.1469-7610.2007.01762.x.

Foster, E. M., & Pearson, E. (2012). Is inclusivity an indicator of quality of care for children with autism in special education? *Pediatrics*, 130 Suppl 2: S179–85. doi: 10.1542/peds.2012-0900P.

Fox, J. J., & Gable, R. A. (2004). Functional behavioral assessment. In R. B. Rutherford, M. M. Quinn, & S. R. Mathur (Eds.), *Handbook of Research in Emotional and Behavioral Disorder* (pp. 143–162). New York, NY: The Guildford Press.

Flippin, M., Reszda, S., & Watson, L. R., (2010). Effectiveness of the picture exchange communication system (PECS) on communication and speech for children with autism spectrum disorders: A meta-analysis. *American Journal of Speech-Language Pathology Research*, Article 1, May, 19(2): 178–195. https://doi.org/10.1044/1058-0360(2010/09-0022). Epub 2010 Feb 24. PMID: 20181849.

Grahame, V., Brett, D., Dixon, L., McConachie, H., Lowry, J., Rodgers J., Steen, N., & Le Couteur, A. (2015). Managing repetitive behaviours in young children with autism spectrum disorder (ASD): Pilot randomised controlled trial of a new parent group intervention. *Journal of Autism and Developmental Disorders*, 45(10): 3168–3182. doi: 10.1007/s10803-015-2474-x. PMID: 26036646.

Gray, C.A., & Garand, J.D. (1993). Social stories: Improving response of students with autism with accurate social information. *Focus on Autistic Behavior*, 8(1): 1–10.

Green, J., Charman, T., McConachie, H., Aldred, C., Slonims, V., Howlin, P., LeCouteur, A., Leadbitter, K., Hudry, K., Byford, S., Barrett, B., Temple, K., Macdonald, W., Pickles, A., & PACT Consortium (2010). PACT Consortium parent-mediated communication-focused treatment in children with autism (PACT): A randomised controlled trial. *Lancet*, 375(9732): 2152–2160.

Gutstein, S. E. (2009). Empowering families through relationship development intervention: An important part of the biopsychosocial management of autism spectrum disorders. *Annals of Clinical Psychiatry*, 21(3): 174–182.

Harrop, C. (2015). Evidence-based, parent-mediated interventions for young children with autism spectrum disorder: The case of restricted and repetitive behaviors. *Autism*, 19(6): 662–672. doi: 10.1177/1362361314545685. Epub 2014 Sep 3.

Havdahl, K. A., von Tetzchner, S., Huerta, M., Lord, C., & Bishop, S. L. (2016) Utility of the Child Behavior Checklist as a screener for autism spectrum disorder. *Autism Research*, 9(1): 33–42. https://doi.org/10.1002/aur.1515.

Holingue, C., Pfeiffer, D., Ludwig, N. N., Reetzke, R., Hong, J. S., Kalb, L.G., & Landa, R. (2023). Prevalence of gastrointestinal symptoms among autistic individuals, with and without co-occurring intellectual disability. *Autism Research*, 16(8): 1609–1818. https://doi.org/10.1002/aur.2972. Epub 2023 Jun 16.

Hyman, S. L., Levy, S. E., Myers, S. M., & Council on Children With Disabilities, Section on Developmental and Behavioral Pediatrics (2020). Identification, evaluation, and management of children with autism spectrum disorder. *Pediatrics*,145(1): e20193447. https://doi.org/10.1542/peds.2019-3447. Epub 2019 Dec 16.

Ibrahim, S. H., Voigt, R. G., Katusic, S. K., Weaver, A. L., & Barbaresi, W. J. (2009) Incidence of gastrointestinal symptoms in children with autism: A population-based study. *Pediatrics*, 124(2): 680–686. https://doi.org/10.1542/peds.2008-2933. Epub 2009 Jul 27.

Ingersoll, B. R., & Wainer, A. L. (2013). Pilot study of a school-based parent training program for preschoolers with ASD. *Autism*, 17(4): 434–448. doi:10.1177/1362361311427155. Epub 2011 Nov 15. PMID: 22087044.

Kasari, C., Rotheram-Fuller, E., Locke, J., & Gulsrud, A. (2012). Making the connection: Randomized controlled trial of social skills at school for children with autism spectrum disorders. *Journal of Child Psychology and Psychiatry*, 53(4): 431–9. doi: 10.1111/j.1469-7610.2011.02493.x. Epub 2011 Nov 26.

Kasari, C., Gulsrud, A., Paparella, T., Hellemann, G., & Berry, K. (2015) Randomized comparative efficacy study of parent-mediated interventions for toddlers with autism. *Journal of Consulting and Clinical Psychology*, 83(3): 554–563. https://doi.org/10.1037/a0039080.

Klass, P., & Costello, E. (2003). *Quirky Kids: Understanding and Helping Your Child Who Doesn't Fit In – When to Worry and When Not to Worry.* New York: Ballantine Books.

Krasny, L., Williams, B. J., Provencal, S., & Ozonoff, S. (2003). Social skills interventions for the autism spectrum: Essential ingredients and a model curriculum. *Child and Adolescent Clinics of North America*,12(1): 107–122.

Kretzmann, M., Shih, W., & Kasari, C. (2015). Improving peer engagement of children with autism on the school playground: A randomized controlled trial. *Behavioral Therapy*, 46(1): 20–8. doi: 10.1016/j.beth.2014.03.006. Epub 2014 Mar 25.

Landry, S. H., Smith, K. E., Swank, P. R., & Miller-Loncar, C.L. (2000). Early maternal and child influences on children's later independent cognitive and social functioning. *Child Development*, 71(2): 358–375. https://doi.org/10.1111/1467-8624.00151.

Laugeson, E. A., Ellingsen, R., Sanderson, J., Tucci, L., & Bates, S. (2014). The ABC's of teaching social skills to adolescents with autism spectrum disorder in the classroom: The UCLA PEERS (®) Program. *Journal of Autism and Developmental Disorders*, 44(9): 2244–2256. doi: 10.1007/s10803-014-2108-8.

Laugeson, E. A., Gantman, A., Kapp, S. K., Orenski, K., & Ellingsen, R. A. (2015). Randomized controlled trial to improve social skills in young adults with autism spectrum disorder: The UCLA PEERS(®) program. *Journal of Autism and Dev Disorders*, 45(12): 3978–3989. https://doi.org/10.1007/s10803-015-2504-8.

Leaf, J. B., Leaf, J. A., Milne, C., Taubman, M., Oppenheiim-Leaf, M., Torres, N., Townley-Cochran, D., Leaf, R., McEachin, J., & Oder, P. (2017). An evaluation of a behaviorally based social skills group for individuals diagnosed with autism spectrum disorder. *Journal of Autism and Developmental Disorders*, 47(2): 243–259. https://doi.org/10.1007/s10803-016-2949-4.

Linstead, E., Dixon, D. R., French, R., Granpeesheh, D., Adams, H., German, R., Powel, A., Stevens, E., Tarbox, J. & Kornack, J. (2017). Intensity and learning outcomes in the treatment of children with autism spectrum disorder. *Behavior Modification*, 41(2): 229–252. https://doi.org/10.1177/0145445516667059. Epub 2016 Sep 21.

Lipkin, P. H., Okamoto, J., Council on Children with Disabilities, & Council on School Health (2015). The Individuals With Disabilities Education Act (IDEA) for children with special educational needs. *Pediatrics*, 136(6): e1650–1662. https://doi.org/10.1542/peds.2015-3409.

Lotfizadeh, A. D., Kazemi, E., Pompa-Craven, P., & Eldevik, S. (2018). Moderate effects of low-intensity behavioral intervention. *Behavior Modification*, 44(1): 92–113. https://doi.org/10.1177/0145445518796204. Epub 2018 Aug 23.

Lord C., Rutter M., DiLavore P. C., Risi S., Gotham K., & Bishop S. (2012). *Autism Diagnostic Observation Schedule – 2nd edition (ADOS-2)*. Torrance, Calif: Western Psychological Services.

Lovaas, O. I. (1987) Behavioral treatment and normal educational and intellectual functioning in young autistic children. *Journal of Consulting and Clinical Psychology*, 55(1), 3–9. https://doi.org/10.1037//0022-006x.55.1.3.

Lovaas, O. I., & Smith, T. A. (1989) A comprehensive behavioral theory of autistic children: Paradigm for research and treatment. *Journal of Behavioral Therapy and Experimental Psychiatry*, 20(1): 17–29. https://doi.org/10.1016/0005-7916(89)90004-9.

Maenner, M. J., Warren, Z., Willams, A. R., Amoakohene, E., Bakian, A. V., Bilder, D. A., Durkin, M. S., Fitzgerald, R. T., Furnier, S. M., Hughes, M. M., Ladd-Acosta, C. M., McArthur, D., Pas, E. T., Salinas, A., Vehorn, A., Williams, S., Esler, A., Grzbowski, A., Hall-Lande, J., Nguyen, R. H. N., Pierce, K., Zahorodny, W., Hudson, A., Hallas, L., Mancilla K. C., Patrick, M., Shenouda, J., Sidwell, K., DiRienzo, M., Gutierrez, J., Spivey, M. H., Lopez, M., Pettygrove, S., Schwenk, Y. D., Washington, A., & Shaw, K.A. (2023). Prevalence and characteristics of autism spectrum disorder among children aged 8 years – Autism and Developmental Disabilities Monitoring Network, 11 Sites, United States, 2020. *Morbidity and Mortality Weekly Report Surveillance Summary*, 72(SS–2): 1–14. https://doi.org/10.15585/mmwr.ss7202a1.

Malow, B. A., Adkins, K. W., Reynolds, A., Weiss, S. K., Loh, A., Fawkes, D., Katz, T., Goldman, A. E., Madduri, N., Hundley, R., & Clemons, T. (2014). Parent-based sleep education for children with autism spectrum disorders *Journal of Autism and Developmental Disorders*, 44(1): 216–228. https://doi.org/10.1007/s10803-013-1866-z.

Mesibov, G. B., Shea, V., & Schopler, E. (2004) *The TEACCH Approach to Autism Spectrum Disorders*. New York, NY: Springer.

Morrison, J. (2014). *DSM-5 Made Easy. The Clinician's Guide to Diagnosis*. New York, NY: Guilford Press.

Nahmias, A. S., Pellecchia, M., Stahmer, A.C., & Mandell, D. S. (2019). Effectiveness of community-based early intervention for children with autism spectrum disorder: A meta-analysis. *Journal of Child Psychology and Psychiatry*, 60(11): 1200–1209. https://doi.org/10.1111/jcpp.13073. Epub 2019 Jun 17.

Oono, I. P., Honey, E. J., & McConachie, H. (2013). Parent-mediated early intervention for young children with autism spectrum disorders (ASD). *Cochrane Database Syst Rev*, 2013(4): CD009774. doi: 10.1002/14651858.CD009774.pub2.

Orinstein, A. J., Helt, M., Troyb, E., Tyson, K. E., Barton, M. L., Eigsti, I-M., Naigles, L., & Fein, D. A. (2014). Intervention for optimal outcome in children and adolescents with a history of autism. *Journal of Developmental and Behavioral Pediatrics*, 35(4): 247–256. https://doi.org/10.1097/DBP.0000000000000037.

Ospina, M. B., Seida, J. K., Clark, B., Karkhaneh, M., Hartling, L., Tjosvold, L., Vandermeer B., & Smith V. (2008). Behavioural and developmental interventions for autism spectrum disorder: A clinical systematic review. *PLoS One*, 3(11): e3755. https://doi.org/10.1371/journal.pone.0003755. Epub 2008 Nov 18.

Otero, T. L., Schatz, R. B., Merrill, A. C., & Bellini, S. (2015). Social skills training for youth with autism spectrum disorders: A follow-up.

Child and Adolescent Psychiatry Clinics of North America, 24(1): 99–115. https://doi.org/10.1016/j.chc.2014.09.002. Epub 2014 Oct 11.

Pagliaro, J. C. (2023). The future of autism and ABA: Predicting outcomes. *Autism Spectrum News.*

Pellecchia, M., Iadarola, S., & Stahmer, A. C. (2019) How meaningful is more? Considerations regarding intensity in early intensive behavioral intervention. *Autism*, 23(5): 1075–1078. https://doi.org/10.1177/1362361319854844. Epub 2019 Jun 6.

Prizant, B., Wetherby, A., Rubin, E., Laurent, A., & Rydell, P. (2006) *The SCERTS Model; A Comprehensive Educational Approach for Children With Autism Spectrum Disorder.* Baltimore, Maryland: Paul H. Brookes Publishing.

Reichow, B., & Volkmar, F. R. (2010). Social skills interventions for individuals with autism: Evaluation for evidence-based practices within a best evidence synthesis framework. *Journal of Autism and Developmental Disorders*, 40(2): 149–166. https://doi.org/10.1007/s10803-009-0842-0. Epub 2009 Aug 5.

Reichow, B., Steiner, A. M., & Volkmar, F. (2013). Cochrane review: Social skills groups for people aged 6 to 21 with autism spectrum disorders (ASD). *Evidence-Based Child Health*, 8(2): 266–315. https://doi.org/10.1002/ebch.1903.

Reichow, B., Hume, K., Barton, E. E., Boyd, B. A., & Cochrane Developmental, Psychosocial and Learning Problems Group (2018). Early intensive behavioral intervention (EIBI) for young children with autism spectrum disorders (ASD). *Cochrane Rev*, 2018(5): CD009260. doi: 10.1002/14651858.CD009260.pub3.

Roane, H. S., Fisher, W. W., & Carr, J. E. (2016). Applied behavior analysis as treatment for autism spectrum disorder. *Journal of Pediatrics*, 175: 27–32. Epub 2016 May 11.

Rogers, S. J., & Dawson, G. (2010) *The Early Start Denver Model for Young Children with Autism: Promoting Language, Learning, and Engagement.* New York, NY: Guilford Press.

Rogers, S. J., Estes, A., Lord, C., Vismara, L., Winter, J., Fitzpatrick, A., Guo, M., & Dawson, G. (2012). Effects of a brief Early Start Denver model (ESDM)-based parent intervention on toddlers at risk for autism spectrum disorders: A randomized controlled trial. *Journal of the American Academy of Child and Adolescent Psychiatry*, 51(10): 1052–1065. doi: 10.1016/j.jaac.2012.08.003. Epub 2012 Aug 28.

Rosenblatt, A. I., & Carbone, P. (2019). *Autism Spectrum Disorders: 2nd Edition: What Every Parent Needs to Know.* Elk Grove Village, IL: American Academy of Pediatrics.

Rutter, M., LeCouteru, A., & Lord, C. (2003). *Autism Diagnostic Interview-Revised (ADI-R)*. Torrance, Calif: Western Psychological Services.

Scahill, L., Bearss, K., Lecavalier, L., Smith, T., Swiezy, N., Aman, M. G., Sukhodolsky, D. G., McCracken, C., Dziura, J., & Johnson, C. (2016). Effect of parent training on adaptive behavior in children with autism spectrum disorder and disruptive behavior: Results of a randomized trial. *Journal of the American Academy of Child and Adolescent Psychiatry*, 55(7): 602–609.e3. doi: 10.1016/j.jaac.2016.05.001. Epub 2016 May 7.

Schreibman, L., Dawson, G., Stahmer, A. C., Landa, R., Rogers, S. J., McGee, G. G., Dasari, C., Ingersoll, B., Kaiser, A. P., Bruinsma, Y., McNerney, E., Wetherby, A., & Halladay, A. (2015). Naturalistic developmental behavioral interventions: Empirically validated treatments for autism spectrum disorder. *Journal of Autism and Developmental Disorders*, 45(8): 2411–2428. https://doi.org/10.1007/s10803-015-2407-8.

Siller, M., & Sigman, M. (2002). The behaviors of parents of children with autism predict the subsequent development of their children's communication. *Journal of Autism and Developmental Disorders*, 32(2): 77–89. https://doi.org/10.1023/a:1014884404276.

Smith, T., & Eikeseth, S. O. (2011). Ivar Lovaas: Pioneer of applied behavior analysis and intervention for children with autism. *Journal of Autism and Developmental Disorders*, 4(3): 375–378. https://doi.org/10.1007/s10803-010-1162-0.

Smith, T., & Iadarola, S. (2015) Evidence base update for autism spectrum disorder. *Journal of Clinical Child and Adolescent Psychology*, 44(6): 897–922. https://doi.org/10.1080/15374416.2015.1077448.

Soke, G. N., Maenner, M. J., Christensen, D., Kurzius-Spencer, M., & Schieve, L. A. (2018). Prevalence of co-occurring medical and behavioral conditions/symptoms among 4-and 8-year-old children with autism spectrum disorder in selected areas of the United States in 2010. *Journal of Autism and Developmental Disorders*, 48(8): 2663–2676. https://doi.org/10.1007/s10803-018-3521-1.

Solomon, R., Van Egeren, L. A., Mahoney, G., Quon Huber, M. S., & Zimmerman, P. (2014). PLAY Project Home Consultation intervention program for young children with autism spectrum disorders: A randomized controlled trial. *Journal of Developmental and Behavioral Pediatrics*, 35(8): 475–485. https://doi.org/10.1097/DBP.0000000000000096.

Strain, P. S., & Bovey, E. H. II. (2011). Randomized, controlled trial of the LEAP model of early intervention for young children with autism spectrum disorders. *Topics in Early Childhood Special Education*, 31(3): 133–154. https://doi.org/10.1177/0271121411408740.

Strain, P. S., & Hoyson, M. (2000). The need for longitudinal, intensive social skill intervention: LEAP follow-up outcomes for children with autism. *Topics in Early Childhood Special Education*, 20(2): 116–122. https://doi.org/10.1177/027112140002000207.

Tamis-LeMonda, C. S., Bornstein, M. H., & Baumwell, L. (2001). Maternal responsiveness and children's achievement of language milestones. *Child Development*, 72(3): 748–767. https://doi.org/10.1111/1467-8624.00313.

Turner-Brown, L., Hume, K., Boyd, B. A., & Kainz, K. (2019) Preliminary efficacy of family implemented TEACCH for toddlers: Effects on parents and their toddlers with autism spectrum disorder. *Journal of Autism and Developmental Disorders*, 49(7): 2685–2698. https://doi.org/10.1007/s10803-016-2812-7.

Verschuur, R., Didden, R., Lang, R., Sigafoos, J., & Huskens, B. (2014). Pivotal response treatment for children with autism spectrum disorders: A systematic review. *Journal of Autism and Developmental Disorders*, 1:34–61. https://doi.org/10.1007/s40489-013-0008-z.

Virues-Ortega, J., Julio, F. M., & Pastor-Barriuso, R. (2013). The TEACCH program for children and adults with autism: A meta-analysis of intervention studies. *Clinical Psychology Reviews*, 33(8): 940–953. https://doi.org/10.1016/j.cpr.2013.07.005. Epub 2013 Jul 24,

Whalon, K. J., Conroy, M. A., Martinez, J. R., & Werch, B. L. (2015). School-based peer-related social competence interventions for children with autism spectrum disorder: A meta-analysis and descriptive review of single case research design studies. *Journal of Autism and Developmental Disorders*, 45(6): 1513–1531.

Wetherby, A. M., Guthrie, W., Woods, J., Schatschneider, C., Holland, R. D., Morgan, L., & Lord, C. (2014). Parent-implemented social intervention for toddlers with autism: An RCT. *Pediatrics*, 134(6): 1084–1093. https://doi.org/10.1542/peds.2014-0757. Epub 2014 Nov 3.

Weitlauf, A. S., McPheeters, M. L., Peters, B., Sathe, N., Travis, R., Aiello, R., Williamson, E., Veenstra-VanderWeele, J., Krishnaswami, S., Jerome, R., & Warren, Z. (2014). *Therapies for children with autism spectrum disorder: Behavioral interventions update*. Rockville, MD: Agency for Healthcare Research and Quality.

Winter, J. (2024). The argument over a long-standing autism intervention. Annals of Medicine. *The New Yorker*.

Yu, Q., Li, E., Li, L., & Liang, W. (2020). Efficacy of interventions based on applied behavior analysis for autism spectrum disorder: A meta-analysis. *Psychiatry Investigation*, 17(5): 432–443. https://doi.org/10.30773/pi.2019.0229.

CHAPTER 5

Attention-Deficit/Hyperactivity Disorder or Just Energetic?

L et us, once again, travel back in time.

Reports of children with difficulty paying attention can be found as early as the 18th century (Barkley & Peters, 2012). In the early 20th century, Sir George Frederic Still published an article in *The Lancet* describing children with "an abnormal defect of moral control." In 1937, psychiatrist Charles Bradley administered benzedrine sulfate, an amphetamine, to children at the Emma Pendleton Bradley Home in Providence, Rhode Island, in an attempt to treat their headaches, and Bradley noticed an unexpected calming effect on their behavior.

During the 20th century several labels were given to describe children who were overly active, distractible and inattentive, including "minimal brain damage," "minimal brain dysfunction," "minimal brain disorder," "learning/behavioral disabilities," and "hyperactivity." In 1952, the first *Diagnostic and Statistical Manual of Mental Disorders* (DSM) was issued by the American Psychiatric Association (APA), but attention-deficit/hyperactivity disorder (ADHD) was not included as a specific mental health diagnosis. In 1955 the Food and Drug Administration (FDA) approved the psychostimulant medication, Ritalin (methylphenidate), and it was in 1968 that the APA officially recognized ADHD as a mental health diagnosis and included the diagnosis of "Hyperkinetic Reaction of Childhood/Hyperkinetic Impulse Disorder" in DSM-II. In 1980 the DSM-III introduced the term "ADD – Attention-Deficit Disorder, with or without hyperactivity," and in 1987, the DSM-III-R changed the diagnosis to ADHD. The DSM-IV distinguished subtypes of ADHD in 1994 (Barkley, 2015, Smith, 2012). During the 1990s, the number of individuals diagnosed with ADHD increased, and new medications became available. In 2000, the DSM-IV-TR continued to include ADHD with subtypes, and in 2013, the DSM-5 included three main presentations of ADHD –

DOI: 10.4324/9781003639121-5

predominantly inattentive, predominantly hyperactive-impulsive, and combined (APA, 2013; Morrison, 2014).

Now, let us introduce some children as described by their parents.

CASE STUDIES

Oliver has just turned five years old. He was adopted when he was four years old. He previously lived in multiple foster homes after Child Services determined that his parents were not able to care for him secondary to their own mental health and intellectual challenges. Oliver seems bright, but he typically has several tantrums each day and he does not listen to instructions. His preschool teacher also reported that he does not follow instructions and is resistant to sharing with the other children. She "hinted" that he may benefit from treatment with medication because he is presenting with features of ADHD.

James is six years old. He has always been active. Even when he was a toddler, he seemed to run instead of walk. When he walks into a room, he touches everything, jumps on furniture and typically cannot sit still long enough to play with his siblings or peers. During preschool, his teacher said he was unable to sit during circle time – one of the assistant teachers needed to hold him and bounce him on her lap. Things seemed to worsen in kindergarten and first grade. James' first grade teacher contacted James' parents and reported that he was unable to function optimally in the classroom and that his behavior was distracting to the other students. Although he was bright, his behavior was having a negative impact on his academic progress – he was unable to complete his schoolwork due to his difficulty staying seated and focused. The teacher suggested that James' parents have him evaluated for ADHD.

Emma is three years old. She began to walk at nine months of age, and she has continued to be very active. She can become restless in a restaurant and sometimes needs a break from sitting. Her parents inquired whether they should have her evaluated for ADHD.

ADHD

Children with ADHD present with a history of multiple symptoms of inattention and/or hyperactivity and impulsivity that interfere with their ability to function in multiple environments, including school. The presentations of ADHD include ADHD inattentive presentation; ADHD hyperactive-impulsive presentation; and ADHD combined presentation (i.e., inattentive and hyperactive-impulsive) (APA, 2013).

Inattention can be characterized by difficulty paying close attention to details and difficulty sustaining attention to schoolwork, chores, or play activities. Because of their limited attention span, children with ADHD do not appear to listen when they are spoken to and often do not follow through on instructions. They can become easily sidetracked and often fail to finish their schoolwork or other tasks and projects. Poor organizational skills are also often observed in these children. This can result in them losing things and appearing forgetful, and can contribute to their failure to complete projects. Children with ADHD may appear to avoid tasks that require them to focus for extended periods of time (APA, 2013; Morrison, 2014).

Hyperactivity and impulsivity can be characterized by a child who frequently moves or fidgets with their hands or feet and has difficulty staying seated and sitting still. Children who are excessively active and impulsive frequently run and climb, not for attention, but because they are unable to regulate/control their movements and activity level. They can therefore have difficulty waiting in lines and waiting their turn during games and in the classroom. Children who are hyperactive are often described as appearing as if they are "driven by a motor." In addition to impulsively moving about, these children can have difficulty monitoring their talking and are often observed to interrupt others and "blurt" out answers before a question has been fully asked (APA, 2013; Morrison, 2014).

Being energetic, however, does not necessarily mean that a child has ADHD. Most children enjoy movement, and young children have limited attention spans. Sometimes adults have limited patience for children who require a great deal of activity and movement – that does not necessarily mean that the child's behavior is abnormal. While a child may have a high energy and activity level that can be challenging during specific activities at home or at school, other factors must be considered when determining an ADHD diagnosis. A qualified professional will assess all aspects of a child's behaviors and actions across multiple settings in order to differentiate between a "high energy" child and a child with ADHD.

CASE STUDIES

Oliver, James and **Emma** all presented with some symptoms of ADHD. They were all referred for evaluations, which included extensive histories, language, cognitive and early learning skill testing, and behavioral rating scales completed by their parents and teachers. Of note, Emma's pediatrician did not feel strongly that Emma's activity level was abnormal for her age, but because of her mother's concerns, Emma was referred for an evaluation.

PREVALENCE

ADHD is reported to be the most common childhood neurobehavioral disorder (Wolraich et al., 2019). Results of the National Interview Survey revealed that the percentage of children diagnosed with ADHD increased from 7% during 1998–2000 to 9% during 2007–2009, with variations reported among different races and ethnicities (Akinbami et al., 2011). Another study covering a 20-year period revealed the prevalence increased from 6.1% in 1997–1998 to 10.2% in 2015–2016 (Xu et al., 2018). A national survey in 2014 reported a median age of diagnosis of seven years, with about one-third of children diagnosed before the age of six (Wolraich, et al., 2019). Data from the most recent National Center for Health Statistics revealed that during 2020–2022, the prevalence of ADHD ("ever diagnosed") was 11.3% in children aged 5 to 17 – 14.5% in boys and 8% in girls (Reuben & Elgaddal, 2024). Additional data was provided by the American Academy of Pediatrics Clinical Guidelines for the Diagnosis, Evaluation, and Treatment of Attention-Deficit/Hyperactivity Disorder in Children and Adolescents. It was reported that ADHD is diagnosed more frequently in males than females, which may be partially related to hyperactivity being more frequently observed in boys. In addition, children who are diagnosed with ADHD are often diagnosed with additional mental health disorders, and boys with ADHD are more likely to exhibit externalizing behaviors including co-morbid diagnoses of oppositional defiant disorder (ODD) and/or conduct disorders. Moreover, hyperactivity and impulsivity tend to decline in adolescence, but inattention typically continues (Wolraich, et al., 2019).

Research has revealed that girls with ADHD are more likely than boys to have a comorbid internalizing condition such as anxiety or depression (Wolraich et al., 2019). In addition to gender differences, ethnic and socioeconomic differences exist, including the following data from the 2020–2023 National Center for Health Statistics: White non-Hispanic children aged 5–17 years were more likely to have ADHD (13.4%) than Black non-Hispanic (10.8%) and Hispanic (8.9%) children. Moreover, the prevalence of ADHD decreased as the level of family income increased. Finally, children with public (14.4%) or private (9.7%) health insurance were more likely to be diagnosed ADHD than children without insurance (6.3%) (Reuben & Elgaddal, 2024).

AUTHORS' COMMENTARY

Why has the prevalence of ADHD increased? An increased awareness regarding the diagnosis, changes in criteria for the diagnosis over time, changes in social norms, and other possible environmental factors may have contributed to a change in the number of children who are diagnosed with ADHD. It is also important to note, however, that children who fidget, daydream, and enjoy running and jumping should not automatically be diagnosed with ADHD.

HOW IS A CHILD DIAGNOSED WITH ADHD?

Similar to other developmental diagnoses, there is no lab or other specific medical test that will determine if a child has ADHD. A diagnosis is based on the child's clinical presentation as well as information from people who have observed the child's behavior. This typically includes parents and teachers but can also include close relatives who spend a great deal of time with the child, daycare providers, therapists, and early intervention staff. The child's physician should confirm that there are no medical conditions that could be impacting the child's behavior – for example, suboptimal nutrition, anemia, or thyroid problems. The evaluation for ADHD should be culturally sensitive and appropriate for the developmental level of the child. The evaluator should review the criteria for ADHD included in the DSM-5. The evaluation typically includes completion of standardized parent and teacher questionnaires, as well as self-report questionnaires, when age-appropriate – for example, **Conners Comprehensive Behavior Rating Scale** (Conners, 2008) and **NICHQ Vanderbilt Assessment Scale** (National Institute for Children's Health Quality, 2002). A screening of a child's communication, cognitive, and academic skills should be included in the assessment. Tools to assess behavior such as the **Behavior Assessment System for Children** and the **Child Behavior Checklist** are not specifically designed to diagnose ADHD, but their results may indicate some features of this diagnosis as well as comorbid conditions (Biederman et al., 2021; Jarratt et al., 2005).

There are also computer-based tests that are sometimes used in the assessment of a child's attention.

Continuous Performance Test (CPT)

Continuous performance tests can assist in measuring sustained attention, selective attention, and also impulsivity. The test typically includes the rapid presentation of a series of visual and/or auditory stimuli during a specific amount of time. The person taking the test must respond by pressing the computer button/bar to the target stimuli and avoid responding to non-target stimuli. Failing to respond to stimuli are considered "omissions", while responding to non-stimuli are considered "commissions." Continuous performance tests have been used a great deal, but reports regarding their efficacy in diagnosing ADHD have been variable, with some studies reporting usefulness, some reporting limitations in sensitivity and/or specificity of the tests, and some reporting an overall limited usefulness in assessing or monitoring symptoms of ADHD (Baggio et al., 2019; Berger et al., 2017; Emser et al., 2018; Gualtieri & Johnson, 2005; Roebuk et al., 2016; Shaked et al., 2020; Tinius, 2003). Some of the research completed on specific CPTs is listed alphabetically below.

Conners CPT – 3rd Edition

Results of a review completed in 2023 by Callan and colleagues revealed that five studies found that the CPT-3 was a weak predictor of ADHD while two found that it was an adequate predictor. Two studies reported that the CPT-3 could differentiate clients with comorbid ADHD/anxiety from ADHD or ADHD from obsessive-compulsive disorder. Finally, one study found that CPT-3 did not differentiate ADHD from autism spectrum disorder (ASD) or comorbid ADHD/ASD (Callan et al., 2023; Callan et al., 2024).

Integrated Visual and Auditory CPT

This CPT has been used in some studies comparing children and adults with ADHD to those with other diagnoses (Tinius, 2003). A study published in China in 2007 indicated that this CPT can assist in making the diagnosis of ADHD, particularly in younger children (Pan et al., 2007).

MOXO-CPT

This test includes auditory and visual distractions that the test taker is required to ignore. Berger and colleagues completed a study using the MOXO-CPT, the results of which revealed that children with ADHD scored lower than their non-ADHD peers in attention, timing, hyperactivity, and impulsivity (Berger et al., 2017).

Qualified Behavior (Qb) Test

This test received approval from the FDA (Ref: K133382). It combines measures of attention (sustained and selective) and impulsivity with motion tracking analysis in evaluating hyperactivity. In a report by Hall and colleagues (2017), clinicians and families completed surveys and interviews regarding their experiences with the QbTest. Results indicated that the QbTest may be a potentially valuable tool to use as part of an early assessment of ADHD. Additional trials of this test were also recommended.

Test of Variables of Attention (TOVA)

This CPT was made commercially available in the early 1990s, with normative data reported for children 6 through 16 years (Greenberg & Waldmant, 1993).

REVIEW OF DIAGNOSTIC METHODS

A recent systemic review of ADHD assessment tools completed by Peterson and colleagues included reviews and analyses of 231 studies in 290 publications. The studies included multiple types of assessment methods, including parent ratings scales, teacher rating scales, self-report scales, neuropsychological testing, machine-learning assisted and virtual reality-based tools, as well as some medical testing, including neuroimaging, EEG studies, and laboratory testing ("blood or urine biomarkers"). The study assessed the degree to which the various assessment tools differentiated children with ADHD from typically developing children. Overall results were variable. Although some assessment tools "showed promising diagnostic performance," it was concluded that a definitive diagnosis of ADHD continues to be based on the judgement of an experienced clinician together with rating scales and input from informants from various settings (Peterson et al., 2024b).

In addition to medical information from the child's physician, direct observation of the child, and results of questionnaires, it is always important for a clinician to obtain detailed family and social histories (you will see this recommendation made several times throughout this book). Family history is often an important piece of a diagnostic puzzle. Has the child's parent(s) or sibling(s) been diagnosed with ADHD or other mental health issues? It is also important to be aware that social stresses can impact a child's behavior and presentation. Is there stress in the family dynamics – for example, a difficult parental separation, chronic illness, domestic violence? Financial and/or living situation stressors? Has the child been the victim of bullying at school? Once it is determined that a child meets criteria for the diagnosis of ADHD and other possible reasons for the child's behavior have been explored, the diagnosis may become definitive.

"COMPLEX ADHD"

In guidelines published in 2020 by a panel of the Society for Developmental and Behavioral Pediatrics, "complex ADHD" was described as:

> ADHD diagnosed in children less than 4 years old or age of presentation greater than 12-years-old; presence of co-existing medical, neurodevelopmental, psychosocial, or mental health conditions that can have a negative impact and complicate the child's ADHD presentation; moderate to severe functional impairment; diagnostic uncertainty; or inadequate response to treatment.
>
> (Barbaresi et al., 2020)

Children with complex ADHD typically require consultation and ongoing follow-up with professionals who have special expertise in the diagnosis.

WHAT CAUSES ADHD?

ADHD is a neurobiological disorder – it is associated with dysregulation of some of the chemicals called neurotransmitters in the brain (specifically, dopamine and noradrenaline). Why are these neurotransmitters regulated differently in children with ADHD? There is not a single answer to that question. However, there are many known factors that can increase a child's risk for this diagnosis. Several specific genetic and nongenetic diagnoses are associated with an increased risk for ADHD. Although a complete list is beyond the scope of this book, some genetic diagnoses that can increase a child's risk for features of ADHD include neurofibromatosis, Tuberous Sclerosis, Smith-Magenis syndrome, Prader Willi syndrome, Fragile X syndrome, inborn errors of metabolism, and various chromosomal abnormalities. Examples of some non-genetic diagnoses that increase a child's risk for features of ADHD include a history of prematurity; in-utero exposure to alcohol (including fetal alcohol syndrome/effects), nicotine, and some illicit substances; lead toxicity; and traumatic brain injury. It is important to note that evaluation for these specific diagnoses is typically not strongly indicated for children whose only presentation is that of ADHD, as these specific diagnoses typically include more findings than just ADHD. Quite often a specific etiology for the diagnosis of ADHD is not identified. Studies have shown that, like other developmental disorders, ADHD is often a multifactorial diagnosis, with both environmental and genetic contributing factors. However, a family history of ADHD, particularly if a child has one or more first degree relatives who have been diagnosed with

ADHD, increases a child's risk for this diagnosis. Heritability ranges have been reported to be between 60% and 90%. With the ability to examine the entire genome, studies have explored certain genetic variations as being associated with an increased risk of ADHD as well as other mental health and neurodevelopmental disorders (Arnet et al., 2023; Demontis et al., 2016; Thapar, 2018).

Researchers have attempted to explore whether there are "brain differences" in children with ADHD. Although data from neuroimaging studies has provided variable results, a recent National Institutes of Health (NIH) study reported that examination of thousands of functional brain images of children and adolescents with and without ADHD from six different data sets revealed atypical interactions between the brain's frontal cortex and the processing centers. The children with ADHD were reported to have "heightened connectivity" between structures deep in the brain (involved with learning and processing information) and structures in the frontal area of the brain (involved with attention and disinhibition). There were reported to be more connections between the two areas, which was found to result in inefficiencies in the connections, described as "altered connectivity." Further research, including studies in diverse populations, was recommended (Norman et al., 2024).

"HELPFUL HINTS" IN DISTINGUISHING AMONG ADHD, AGE-APPROPRIATE BEHAVIORS, AND OTHER DIAGNOSES

If a child's parents report that the child is overly active and does not listen to instructions, but the child's teachers and/or daycare providers have not consistently reported that the child's distractibility, limited attention span, or high activity level and impulsivity have negatively impacted on the child's functioning at school/daycare, then the diagnosis of ADHD is less likely. If there has only been one teacher that has had concerns about the child's ability to focus, this could be related to the specific style of that teacher or classroom composition. However, if teachers in lower grades did not express concerns, but the child's teachers in a higher grade expressed concerns, it is also possible that the child's difficulty focusing became more apparent when the academic demands and need for focusing became greater (make sure a learning disability is ruled out, but we will get to that later). However, a typical history is that several teachers have observed the child's difficulty paying attention at school.

A child's attention span is typically at the same level as their cognitive skills. Therefore, if a child's intellectual/cognitive level is at a two- or three-year-old level, their activity level and attention span would be expected to be similar to those of a typical two- or three-year-old child.

Children who appear more energetic than their peers, but have no problem functioning in group activities, are unlikely to have ADHD.

If a child has experienced trauma, they may demonstrate some symptoms similar to those of children with ADHD. Although some of the ADHD treatments may be helpful, the underlying history of trauma, including treatment for posttraumatic stress disorder (PTSD), is a priority (see Chapter 11). Children with anxiety can also present with difficulty focusing – if a child is constantly worried, they will struggle to pay attention to schoolwork and other tasks (see Chapter 8).

Children who have language delays and children who have hearing impairments may appear to have short attention spans. If a child is unable to understand instructions and conversations or unable to fully hear what is being said, their ability to pay attention will be compromised. Difficulty expressing themself could result in frustration and acting out, possibly appearing as impulsivity or hyperactivity.

If a child's difficulty listening to instructions appears more related to the child's behavior – for example, noncompliance, oppositionality, or attention seeking – the child may be presenting with an alternative behavioral diagnosis.

It is also important to note that many children with a definitive diagnosis of ADHD often meet criteria for additional diagnoses.

Let us return to Oliver, James, and Emma.

CASE STUDIES

As part of **Oliver's** evaluation, it was revealed that he had a history of physical and emotional abuse. Oliver's language and early learning skills were tested to be within normal limits. Although Oliver had a history of features of ADHD, it was felt that his primary diagnosis was more likely PTSD.

During **James'** evaluation he required a great deal of redirection. Results of parent and teacher questionnaires revealed multiple features of ADHD, and it was felt that he met full criteria for this diagnosis.

Results of **Emma's** evaluation revealed age-appropriate skills and age-appropriate ability to follow directions and attend to tasks. It was not felt that she met criteria for the diagnosis of ADHD.

OTHER BEHAVIORS AND DIAGNOSES OBSERVED WITH INCREASED FREQUENCY IN CHILDREN WITH ADHD

Oppositional Behaviors: Children with ADHD are at increased risk for behavioral problems. In addition to their features of ADHD, they can demonstrate a limited frustration tolerance, poorer coping skills, and a higher frequency of noncompliant and oppositional behaviors. A diagnosis of ODD can co-occur with ADHD.

- **Poor emotional and behavioral self-regulation**: Children with ADHD often have more difficulty regulating and controlling their behavior and emotions compared to children without an ADHD diagnosis.
- **Sleep problems**: Children with ADHD are more likely to experience sleep difficulties – for example, difficulty falling asleep and difficulty staying asleep, compared to children without developmental-behavioral diagnoses.
- **Anxiety**: It is important to attempt to determine if a child's inattention is a child's primary problem or related to anxiety. However, children with ADHD are considered to be at an increased risk for anxiety related issues, and the diagnosis of an anxiety disorder can co-occur with ADHD.
- **Other mental health diagnoses**: It is important for children with ADHD to be assessed and monitored for other mental health diagnoses, including PTSD, anxiety, depression, ODD, and mood disorders.

TREATMENTS FOR ADHD

Treatment of ADHD should address a child's specific symptoms of ADHD and the functional challenges associated with the diagnosis. Goals should target improving the parents' and child's ability to understand and manage their symptoms, improve the child's functioning, decrease co-morbidities, and hopefully improve long-term outcomes. As with other developmental diagnoses, behavioral and educational supports are paramount. In addition, it can also be beneficial to combine these interventions and supports with pharmacological treatment as needed.

Initial results of an important multimodal treatment study of ADHD (MTA) published in 1999 did not reveal a significant improvement in outcome comparing medication and behavioral therapy with medication alone (MTA Cooperative Group, 1999). However, a re-analysis of the MTA, which combined parent and teacher ratings of symptoms, did report improved outcomes for the combination of behavioral therapy with medication (Jensen et al., 2002). A recent systematic review of ADHD treatments completed by Peterson and colleagues included 312 studies in 540 publications. Treatments included medications, psychosocial interventions, parent support, nutrition and supplements, neurofeedback, neurostimulation, physical exercise, complementary medicine, school interventions, and provider approaches. Results revealed that "several treatments improved ADHD symptoms." Treatment with medication had the strongest evidence for addressing symptoms and improving outcomes but was also associated with "adverse events" (Peterson et al., 2024a)

Before initiating treatment for children with ADHD, an important first step is to provide the family, and the child if age-appropriate, with information about the diagnosis. In addition to parent groups and written and online information, there are books designed for young children and adolescents that can assist them in understanding the challenges associated with this diagnosis.

AUTHORS' COMMENTARY

Although the benefit from pharmacological/medication treatment for children with ADHD is widely accepted, we feel that behavioral and educational approaches are vitally important components of the treatment plan for these children. It has typically been our policy to explore the child's and family's history in depth and first initiate counseling and educational supports, particularly in younger children, before initiating a trial of treatment with medication.

MEDICATIONS

Psychostimulant medications/stimulants have been used for decades for children with ADHD and are typically the first line of medication treatment. Psychostimulant medications typically work by increasing the availability of the neurotransmitter dopamine. Names of some psychostimulant medications include methylphenidate, dexmethylphenidate, dexadrine, amphetamine salts, and lisdexamfetamine. Psychostimulant medications are considered "controlled substances," as they have the potential to be misused. These medications are often available in short acting forms, which typically need to be taken more than once a day, or long-acting/

slow-release/extended-release forms. The effect of a psychostimulant medication is typically observed on the first day it is taken. Psychostimulant medications should not be given in the evening or at night, as they can interfere with a child's ability to fall asleep. Some of the potential side effects of psychostimulant medication include decreased appetite (most common); weight loss; jitteriness; sleep problems; headaches; tics, which can be precipitated in a child who is predisposed to tics or can worsen in a child with a tic disorder; and emotional changes/negative behavioral responses. Starting at a low dose of medication and increasing gradually, while also increasing the caloric density of meals and snacks, can sometimes help lessen some of the potential side effects. Children who are treated with psychostimulant medications require frequent follow-up of their growth parameters. Additional side effects that can require a change in medication type include an increase in anxiety and/or irritability. A limited number of ADHD medications have been approved for use in preschool-aged children, and potential side effects in these young children may include repetitive movements, social withdrawal, and decreased energy (Wolraich et al., 2019). Preschoolers are also at an increased risk for a decline in appetite and poor weight gain and therefore require even more careful follow-up of their growth parameters.

Misuse of psychostimulant medications has been reported, including "sharing" of medication with family members or friends or use of psycho-stimulants as a performance enhancer for academics or sports. Overdose is possible and more recently "street psychostimulants" have sometimes included illicit substances that can be potentially fatal. Finally, stimulant medications carry a "black box" warning because of their potential for abuse and psychological and/or physical dependence. However, so far the use of psychostimulant medication to treat ADHD has not been found to be associated with future substance use; although it has been reported that having a diagnosis of ADHD can increase a child's risk of problems during adulthood, which may include substance use (Klein et al., 2012; Lee et al., 2011; Levy et al., 2014).

There are also nonstimulant medications that are approved for treatment of ADHD. Atomoxetine works by inhibiting the neurotransmitter chemicals norepinephrine and serotonin. Unlike stimulants, it does not have to be taken early in the day. However, the effect of the medication may not be observed until it has been taken for a few weeks. Potential severe negative side effects are rare, however suicidal thoughts and liver abnormalities are included as potential risks.

ADHD medications are "sympathomimetic" agents – that is, they have an effect on the sympathetic nervous system, the part of your nervous system that speeds up your heard rate, delivers blood to areas of your body that need more oxygen, and controls other responses your body has in response to "danger." ADHD medications typically have effects on the neurotransmitters dopamine and/or noradrenaline, which can increase heart rate and blood pressure. Monitoring of a child's heart rate and blood pressure is part of the ongoing care of children who are prescribed ADHD medications. Over the years, there have been concerns that treatment with ADHD medications, particularly psychostimulants, may increase the risk for cardiovascular problems. Several randomized controlled studies revealed no significant short-term cardiovascular effects, although increased heart rate and blood pressure while taking medication has been reported (Hennissen et al., 2017). It is notable that in February 2005, sale of a particular extended-release amphetamine salt was temporarily suspended in Canada in order to explore reports of isolated heart-related deaths in individuals who had been taking this medication (the sale of the same short acting amphetamine salt was not suspended). The suspension was discontinued in August 2005. Results of a meta-analysis completed in 2022 suggested no significant association between ADHD medication use and the risk of cardiovascular disease across age groups, although:

> a modest risk increase could not be ruled out, especially for the risk of cardiac arrest or tachyarrhythmias. Further investigation is warranted for the cardiovascular risk in female patients and patients with preexisting cardiovascular disease as well as long term risks associated with ADHD medication use.
>
> (Zhang et. al., 2022)

A subsequent case-control study completed by Zhang and colleagues included 278,027 children and adults. Results revealed that "longer cumulative duration of ADHD medication use was associated with an increased risk of cardiovascular disease, particularly hypertension and arterial disease, compared with nonuse." Regarding specific medications, the study suggested that "increasing cumulative durations of methylphenidate and lisdexamfetamine use were associated with incident CVD (cardiovascular disease), while the associations for atomoxetine were statistically significant only for the first year of use" (Zhang et al., 2024).

Another nonstimulant medication, guanfacine, lowers blood pressure by activating certain central nervous system receptors. It is available in short acting form, which is typically a twice a day dosing, and long acting/extended release, which is given once a day (this is the preparation that was initially approved for treatment of ADHD). Potential side effects include sleepiness/lethargy, dry mouth, fatigue, and constipation; some of the less common side effects include hair loss, low heart rate, low blood pressure, increased appetite and weight gain, dizziness, and irritability. There is also a potential for a "rebound" increase in blood pressure if the medication is discontinued abruptly.

Similar to guanfacine, clonidine also lowers blood pressure by activating certain central nervous system receptors. It is shorter acting than guanfacine and often more sedating and is therefore sometimes used to treat difficulty falling asleep. There is a longer acting form of the medication that is typically given twice a day. Potential side effects can include dizziness, sleepiness, dry mouth, headache, and low blood pressure; some of the less common side effects include constipation, nausea, and weight gain or loss.

AUTHOR'S COMMENTARY

It is standard of care to monitor all children's growth parameters and their cardiovascular status, including heart auscultation, heart/pulse rate, and blood pressure, with more frequent monitoring recommended for children taking medication to treat ADHD. Regarding children with a history of heart problems, including those with congenital heart disease, clearance from the child's cardiologist before beginning treatment with medication was part of our practice.

BEHAVIORAL AND EDUCATIONAL THERAPY/TREATMENT OF ADHD

Behavioral therapies, as well as behavioral training for parents and school personnel, are accepted treatments for children with ADHD (Evans et al., 2014; Evans et al., 2018; Shepard & Dickstein, 2009; Webster-Stratton et al., 2011; Wolraich et al., 2019). However, the data regarding some training programs (for example, social skills training) have not consistently shown efficacy (Evans et al., 2018).

PARENT TRAINING

Behavioral Strategies to implement at home are included in the Handout for Caregivers at the end of this chapter. However, it is important for clinicians to understand the importance of parent education and training as part of behavior management strategies. It can be beneficial to teach caregivers behavior modification techniques and home scheduling and environmental modifications, with a goal of improving a child's functioning within and outside of the home. An understanding of positive reinforcement for appropriate behaviors and appropriate consequences for unacceptable behaviors are important techniques for all parents and caregivers, but likely hold even more importance for caregivers of children with ADHD.

It has been reported that parent training in behavioral techniques can be effective in reducing problematic behaviors and improving adaptive skills for children with ADHD and other behavioral challenges (Wolraich et al., 2019). Parent training in behavior management strategies is one of the first types of interventions that may be recommended to address behavioral issues in children with ADHD, particularly for younger children. A multi-site study of methylphenidate treatment in preschool-aged children revealed that symptoms improved after parent training in behavior management alone – without medication (Chuang & Cooper, 2006).

AUTHORS' COMMENTARY

Behavioral interventions and supports can be beneficial for children with ADHD. However, it is also important to note that many behavioral interventions for home and school, including parent and educator training, can also benefit children who may not meet criteria for ADHD.

There may be some challenges in implementing behavioral strategies at home, including parent training – for example, parental resistance, financial constraints, family schedules, and lack of resource availability. Although we often recommend behavioral supports and training as a first line of treatment for children with ADHD and other behavioral challenges, particularly for younger children, sometimes there are obstacles that make this difficult. Difficulties accessing parent supports and/or implementing behavioral strategies at home can sometimes result in a clinician feeling that, after assessing the risks of the child's challenges, it makes sense to initiate a very cautious trial of treatment with medication with very close follow-up, while continuing to explore ways to access behavioral supports for the child.

CLASSROOM/SCHOOL ACCOMMODATION AND INTERVENTIONS

If a child with ADHD qualifies for an individualized education program (IEP), their IEP should include accommodations to address their features of ADHD. If a child who has been diagnosed with ADHD does not qualify for an IEP, creation of a 504 Accommodation Plan is recommended, as the diagnosis ADHD meets criteria for a disability based on Section 504 of the Rehabilitation Act of 1973 and the Americans with Disabilities Act. Classroom-based behavior management techniques are well-accepted interventions for children with ADHD, with "large effect sizes in a very large number of studies conducted in schools" (Wolraich et al., 2019). In the 2019 American Academy of Pediatrics Clinical Practice Guideline for the Diagnosis, Evaluation, and Treatment of Attention-Deficit/Hyperactivity Disorder in Children and Adolescents, it was stated that children with ADHD have a disability and should therefore qualify for a service plan under Section 504, which should include academic and behavioral interventions and supports (Wolraich et al., 2019). Examples of some interventions and accommodations, some of which may be included in a student's 504 Accommodation Plan include the following.

- Have a clearly defined schedule and routine with as much predictability and structure as possible.
- Clearly specify rules, expectations, and instructions. Instructions and interventions should be given in brief, understandable sentences and in a non-threatening manner. Instructions should also be given both before and after distribution of materials.
- A classroom schedule and rules can be posted in the classroom, with additional personal copies for the student.
- Provide immediate and consistent feedback on behavior and redirection to task, while providing positive reinforcement for appropriate behavior and work completion/accuracy.
- Establish reasonable, meaningful, and consistent consequences for both compliance and noncompliance.
- Provide the student with frequent opportunities for direct supervision and feedback from the teacher. Develop a "private signal" system with the teacher to gently remind the student when off task or acting inappropriately.
- Provide the student with preferential seating in order to maximize teacher cues and minimize environmental distractions, such as being near open doors leading to corridors, windows opening to the playgrounds, etc., to promote task focus.

- Ensure frequent parent–teacher contact with an assignment or agenda book to coordinate home and school efforts.
- Develop a system of positive reinforcement and feedback to focus as much as possible on shaping appropriate behaviors and interactions. If possible, identify an academic strength or another skill that will allow the student to act as a peer tutor to boost self-esteem and confidence.
- Break down assignments into smaller components and provide frequent feedback on progress.
- Intersperse work period with short periods of physical activity or stretching.
- Give classroom responsibilities, such as being a "helper", to provide an "escape-valve" when the student appears overwhelmed or frustrated.
- Emphasize quality rather than quantity of work; modify the length of a child's assignments/homework.
- Allow the student extra time to complete tests and assignments.
- Provide the student with an area with minimal distractions for test-taking.
- Encourage the use of highlighters and the practice of arranging papers in columns and rows to help to provide structure and assist in organization; teach the habit of reviewing materials and finding and correcting errors.
- Preview upcoming events/transitions.

LET US DISCUSS EXECUTIVE FUNCTION DEFICITS

Executive function includes a group of cognitive processes that are needed to control and monitor an individual's behavior. Examples of executive functions include working memory, cognitive flexibility, the ability to pay attention, and the ability to inhibit impulses. A weakness in executive functioning is often a feature of the diagnosis of ADHD. There are interventions designed to address these executive function weaknesses, although not all of them have been proven to be efficacious based on research studies.

"Working memory" is the term use to describe the cognitive system for holding, processing, and manipulating information. Deficits in working memory can be an area of weakness for children with ADHD. Formal working memory training has not been shown to definitively generalize to overall improvements in a child's performance and functioning (Chacko et al., 2014). However, it appears appropriate for some teaching techniques targeting working memory to be included in a child's program – for example, providing the student with written directions in addition to oral directions and teaching how to highlight important information, appropriate notetaking skills, and outlining.

Initiation is the ability to begin tasks/projects. Initiation can also be challenging for children with ADHD. It may therefore be helpful to break down assignments into small "chunks", as beginning a shorter task (the first "chunk") may be less overwhelming.

Difficulty focusing and paying attention are hallmarks of ADHD. Try to eliminate as many distractions as possible when a child is trying to focus on a project, and try to avoid overstimulating environments

To assist a child with their time management, it may be helpful to create schedules, calendars, planners, and to-do lists. Dividing tasks into immediate, intermittent, and extended deadlines with a calendar of when each piece/chunk of the project should be completed may make the entire project feel less overwhelming.

Attention shifting means the ability to change from one activity to another. Planning transitions, for example, with five-minute warnings can be a helpful strategy to improve a child's ability to transition to a new activity.

Organizational skills can be challenging for children with ADHD. Organizational skills training involves teaching how to organize learning materials, track assignments, and plan work completion. It has been reported that there is some evidence that organizational skills training can be beneficial for older elementary-aged children and adolescents with ADHD (Wolraich et al., 2019). Examples of some general strategies for parents and educators to help facilitate organizational skills include minimizing clutter, color-coding materials, creating templates for writing assignments, and establishing a daily routine.

PEER-RELATIONSHIP TRAINING

It is not uncommon for children with ADHD to experience social challenges. Impulsivity and overactivity can be difficult for a child's peers to tolerate. Some children with ADHD may also have difficulty understanding age-appropriate social behaviors. Social groups focusing on appropriate social behaviors are sometimes provided as part of a school program, and also sometimes as part of social skills groups outside of school. During these groups children are taught how to more successfully interact with their peers. Management of social skills challenges can also be part of a child's individual behavior plan at school or part of their counseling outside of school. There have been studies supporting the efficacy of behavioral interventions directed at peer interaction in social settings, such as at camp or school, i.e., the interventions appear more successful when they are implemented in the social environments in which the child's difficulty typically occurs (Wolraich et al., 2019).

ADDITIONAL AND "ALTERNATIVE" THERAPIES AND INTERVENTIONS

Although the foundations of treatment for symptoms of ADHD include medication and educational and behavioral strategies, additional treatments are sometimes sought out by parents and practitioners. Some additional treatments that have been marketed as potentially helpful for children with ADHD include the following (in alphabetical order).

Cannabidiol Oil

The use of cannabidiol in benefitting children with ADHD is currently considered anecdotal and has not been studied scientifically (Wolraich et al., 2019).

Dietary Modifications and Supplements

Although there has been a great deal of press over the years regarding specific diets that either worsen features of ADHD or alleviate them, results of multiple studies have not resulted in a strong connection between diet and ADHD. An exception is Omega-3 fatty acid supplement which has been shown to be helpful for some individuals with ADHD (Wilens et al., 2017). It is notable that the importance of a well-balanced, healthy diet for all children, including those with ADHD, is universally accepted.

Digital Interventions: "Brain Games"/"Brain Training"

In the current "digital age," there have been products, typically via computer, tablet, or smartphone, that have been publicized as adjunctive treatments for ADHD. Of note, some digital, game-like products have been approved by the FDA. Although these interventions present with a game-like design and format, they differ from games played for entertainment. The products are reportedly designed to improve attention, processing speed, cognitive flexibility, working memory, visual-spatial skills, and/or inhibitory control. More research is needed, but based on studies to date it appears that although children who play these games may improve their "scores" over time – i.e., show an improvement in their ability to focus on the game – so far these skills have not been shown to carry over into improvements in "real life." No definitive negative side effects have been reported, but children can become frustrated with digital game and programs; in addition, sometimes digital exposure can precipitate headaches. It is also important to note that FDA clearance does not necessarily mean that the games are effective (Cortese et al., 2014; Hollis et al., 2017; Kollins et al., 2020; Oldrati et al., 2020). The benefits and risks of these types of programs require further investigation.

AUTHORS' COMMENTARY

It is not unusual for a parent to report that they do not feel that their child has ADHD because the child can focus and pay attention to video games for hours. But think about it, video games continually and rapidly change their visual images – so a child only focuses on the picture on the screen for an exceptionally short amount of time before it changes. Therefore, being able to "focus" on video games does not rule out ADHD.

Exercise

Physical exercise is important for everyone, and particularly children with ADHD. Regular exercise can improve mood and concentration. Some physical activities may be more challenging for children with ADHD. For example, a "team" of four-year-old children running full speed toward a soccer ball may be overwhelming for a child who has difficulty handling overstimulation. Swimming, however, may be more "therapeutic." In addition, under the supervision of an understanding and well-trained instructor, some activities such as martial arts and horseback riding may be helpful in facilitating a child's attentional skills.

External Trigeminal Nerve Stimulation (eTNS)

Although there was a study reporting benefits of eTNS in 30 individuals (McGough et al., 2019), the efficacy of this treatment is currently not felt to be definitive, and eTNS is currently not considered a recommended treatment of ADHD (Wolraich et al., 2019).

Music and Art-Based Therapies

The arts, including visual arts, music, and theater, can provide powerful contributions to an individual's well-being and creativity. Similar to exercise, the arts often prove to be positive experiences for children with ADHD. Both the performing and visual arts can provide creative outlets that can be beneficial to a child's self-esteem, assist the child with learning to focus and pay attention, and also expose the child to other children with similar interests.

Neurofeedback

Biofeedback is a mind-body technique that can be used to gain control of some bodily functions such as heart rate and breathing. Neurofeedback is a type of biofeedback that uses an electroencephalogram (EEG) to measure brain activity. Individuals are trained to produce brain waves thought to be more similar to individuals without ADHD. Although there are mixed opinions on this therapy, overall, it has not been shown to reduce long-term symptoms of ADHD.

AUTHORS' COMMENTARY

Parents should be advised to exercise caution when they are presented with new therapies or treatments for ADHD, particularly if the therapy is reported to "cure" ADHD and possibly treat multiple other diagnoses. Parents should keep in mind that any proposed therapy that is time consuming and expensive should be approached with caution and should be discussed with their child's physician, school staff, therapists, etc.

CASE STUDIES

Oliver was referred to a counselor with expertise in working with children with a history of trauma. His symptoms gradually showed improvement, but at the request of his counselor, a 504 Accommodation Plan was implemented in school based on his diagnosis of PTSD. The Plan included regularly scheduled meetings with the school adjustment counselor.

James was provided with a 504 Accommodation Plan in school that included preferential seating, breaking down of instructions, and movement breaks. James's parents also met with a counselor to help implement appropriate strategies at home. When James was in the second grade he was started on a treatment of psychostimulant medication.

Emma did well at preschool and excelled in motor activities. She enjoyed participating in dance and soccer as extracurricular activities. Her ability to sit was not reported to be problematic during elementary school.

AUTHORS' COMMENTARY

What Does the Future Hold for Children with ADHD?

Multiple studies have reported that children with ADHD are at an increased risk for many adverse adult outcomes, including psychological/mental health, family, social, occupational, and legal problems (Harstad et al., 2022). Despite the validity of these data, we feel it is important to also include our experiences with so many children with ADHD who worked through their challenges, and with the support of their families and access to resources, had successful college, employment, and future family experiences. We therefore recommend "cautious optimism" when working with this diverse and fascinating group of children and their families.

Similar to other neurodevelopmental and mental health diagnoses, we feel that a multidisciplinary approach is beneficial for children with ADHD – both in school and outside counseling, including close medical follow-up with the child's primary care physician, and sometimes including a consulting developmental pediatrician, psychiatrist, or neurologist. Working as a team with the child's teacher(s), school psychologist, and sometimes the school behavioral specialist, together with the child and their family members, can enable coordination of an optimal therapeutic program to address the child's weaknesses and facilitate their strengths.

HANDOUT FOR CAREGIVERS

Attention-Deficit/Hyperactivity Disorder (ADHD)

Children with ADHD present with multiple symptoms of inattention and/or hyperactivity and impulsivity that interfere with their ability to function in multiple environments, including school and home.

Examples of inattention include difficulty paying attention to schoolwork, chores, and play activities. Because of their limited attention span, children with ADHD do not appear to listen when they are spoken to and often do not follow through on instructions. They can become easily sidetracked and often fail to finish schoolwork or other tasks and projects. Poor organizational skills are also often observed in these children, and this can result in them losing things and appearing forgetful, and can contribute to their failure to complete projects. Children with ADHD may appear to avoid tasks that require them to focus for extended periods of time.

A child with hyperactivity and impulsivity frequently moves or fidgets with their hands or feet and has difficulty staying seated and sitting still. Children who are excessively active and impulsive frequently run and climb, not for attention, but because they are unable to regulate/control their movements and activity level. They can therefore have difficulty waiting in lines and waiting their turn during games and in the classroom. Children who are hyperactive are often described as appearing as if they are "driven by a motor." In addition to impulsively moving about, these children can have difficulty monitoring their talking and are often observed to interrupt others and "blurt" out answers before a question has been fully asked (APA, 2013; Morrison, 2014).

Being energetic, however, does not necessarily mean that a child has ADHD. Most children enjoy movement, and young children have limited attention spans. Sometimes adults have limited patience for children who require a great deal of activity and movement – that does not necessarily mean that the child's behavior is abnormal.

Treatments and Interventions

Although there are many interventions marketed for treatment of ADHD, the hallmark treatments/interventions include behavioral supports, both at school and outside of school, and medication when appropriate.

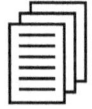

"Helpful Hints" for Caregivers

- Provide a structured environment and create a schedule – i.e., specific time periods for waking up, bedtime, chores, homework, playtime, TV time, meals, etc. Explain any changes in routine ahead of time so that the child understands and can anticipate the changes.
- Set up clear and concise rules of behavior for the family, including your child, but try to keep the number of rules to a minimum. Rules, as well as consequences for breaking them, and rewards for appropriate behavior can be written down and posted in a prominent place. If a rule is broken, consequences should follow every time. If your child behaves appropriately, reward them often. Be firm on setting limits, but give plenty of love and affection too.
- Give instructions as simply and clearly as possible, demonstrating if necessary. Ask your child to repeat instructions back to you, then praise them when they respond correctly. Do not give more than one or two instructions at a time. If a task is difficult, break it into smaller parts and teach each part separately.
- Sometimes repeating messages, directions, requests, etc., too many times is inefficient and can create a variety of unpleasant behaviors in the family. To stop this ineffective process, try the following: Say what you need to say, but say it once, briefly, clearly, completely, firmly, and calmly. Follow through with a logical consequence or restructuring technique. Act, don't "nag."
- Provide your child with his own "special" quiet spot without distractions in which to do academic work or quiet work. Face the desk toward a blank wall, minimize clutter, and avoid bright, distracting colors or patterns in décor. Remember that the child has difficulty filtering out unnecessary stimulation.
- Try to keep your child's stimulation as low as possible. Have him play with one child at a time, involve him in one activity at a time, remove needless background noise such as the radio or TV, and put unused toys, games etc., out of sight.
- Help your child keep his room and play area neat and clean. Provide him with shelves and/or marked boxes for toys. Have a place for everything and help your child learn to keep everything in its place.
- Provide supervision by being physically near the child.
- Allow the child choices within the limits you have set. Help them develop their initiative and self-control and provide a sense of personal influence.
- Use a timer with small chores in order to help give your child a sense of passing time.

- Help your child find avenues of self-expression that will help them express their wants in an acceptable, useful manner. Children sometimes use misbehavior to communicate. Teach appropriate verbal communication skills. Ask yourself, "What does my child want to have happen as a result of this behavior?" and help them search for other ways to gain it.
- Sometimes your child's behavior may be irritating. However, should you become excessively angry, your effectiveness with your child will be greatly reduced. Strive to keep your voice quiet and slow when managing your child's behavior.

Common Questions

Can medication help a child even though he has not been diagnosed with ADHD?

Medications that help children with ADHD improve their ability to pay attention and focus are not necessarily only effective for children with ADHD. Treatment with stimulant medications could potentially help many people improve their ability to pay attention, but that alone would not necessarily be an appropriate reason for treatment. For example, an adolescent who "heard" that treatment with a stimulant medication would help them to focus better in class and study for longer hours would not be an appropriate person for treatment. There are some individuals who are treated for alternative mental health diagnoses who may also have "features of ADHD"; treating them with an ADHD medication would be their physician's decision, particularly if the medication may improve their functioning.

Can my two-year-old child be diagnosed with ADHD?

In the past, a child was not able to be definitively diagnosed with ADHD until he was at least six years old. However, the American Academy of Pediatrics (AAP) later confirmed that children as young as four years old could be diagnosed and treated for ADHD. Although children with ADHD often have histories of features of this diagnosis at a young age, two years old is considered too young for a definitive diagnosis of ADHD (Wolraich et al., 2019). To diagnose a child with ADHD at such a young age could be a disservice – at this developmental stage children are often active and just learning to focus for longer periods of time.

Does a diagnosis of ADHD qualify a child for an individualized education plan?

ADHD is considered a medical/"health" diagnosis, which typically qualifies a student for a 504 Accommodation Plan under Section 504 of the Rehabilitation Act of 1973 (Office of the Assistant Secretary for Administration and Management, 1973). A 504 Plan includes accommodations such as modifications to the environment, modifications to a child's instruction, and/or changes to the curriculum. For example, a student with ADHD may be allowed to take tests in a room with less distractions; allowed extra time to complete assignments; provided with seating that is closer to the teacher and away from distractions such as the window; and allowed to take breaks during class time when he appears more fidgety and less focused. Although there are individual cases when an individualized education program (IEP) will be created based on a child's social emotional challenges and/or academic difficulties, the diagnosis of ADHD does not necessarily qualify a student for special education services, i.e., an IEP.

Since my child has ADHD, there is a neurological reason for some of the behaviors; so, should I still discipline/punish them for the negative behaviors that "are not their fault"?

Although it is true that children with ADHD are often not acting out purposefully, they must still learn skills to regulate and monitor their behavior. However, that does not mean that "punishing" a child for their unacceptable behavior is necessary. First, remember that your child's behavior may be immature, i.e., likely more similar to a child who is younger than his current age. Your response to their behavior should therefore be more similar to your response to a younger child with similar behaviors. First you can attempt to figure out a reason for the behavior – is your child frustrated because a task is too overwhelming or difficult? Once your child is calm, try to teach appropriate responses to frustrating or overwhelming tasks or situations. Acknowledge how difficult it is, but also teach that inappropriate behaviors are unacceptable and together you must learn to express feelings in more appropriate ways.

Can my child who has been diagnosed with autism spectrum disorder also have ADHD?

Impulsivity, hyperactivity and inattention are not uncommonly observed in children with ASD. The most recent *Diagnostic and Statistical Manual of Mental Disorders* (DSM) does not exclude children with ASD as also being able to meet criteria for the diagnosis of ADHD. Behavioral strategies that are provided for children with ADHD can also often be helpful for children with other diagnoses, including autism spectrum disorder (ASD). Similarly, medications that are used to treat children with ADHD can also be helpful in treating the symptoms of ADHD in children with other diagnoses, including ASD. However, caution should always be used and close medical monitoring is essential, as there is a risk that certain ADHD medications may worsen agitation and/or anxiety in children with ASD.

Can a child have symptoms of ADHD only at home and not at school?
If symptoms of ADHD are not observed at school, then most often this rules out this diagnosis. However, implementing behavioral strategies that are helpful for children with ADHD can often be beneficial in addressing these types of behaviors at home even if a child is not definitively diagnosed with ADHD.

My child can focus on building with connecting blocks for extended periods of time. He also spends hours focusing on video games? Does this mean he cannot have ADHD?
Visual changes in video games occur in rapid succession and are therefore often reported to be an activity that can appear to sustain the attention of children with ADHD. In addition, hands-on activities that "keep moving," such as connecting blocks to make buildings and designs, also have a reputation for keeping a child with ADHD focused much longer than many other activities.

Does treatment with psychostimulant medication only work for children with ADHD?
Treatment with psychostimulant medication can improve a person's ability to focus and pay attention, whether or not they have ADHD.

As my child grows, will an increase in the dose of medication be needed?
As a child grows, it is likely that their dose of medication will need to be increased in order for it to continue to be effective. However, many children begin to learn strategies to improve their ability to focus, so sometimes a child can remain on the same dose for an extended period of time, even if they have gained weight. Your child's behavior and feedback from their teacher will be considered by your child's treating physician to determine if an increase in dose of medication is needed.

I noticed recently that my child has been speaking disrespectfully to me. Should I ask the pediatrician to increase their dose of medication?
Although medication can help a child better regulate their behavior, before requesting an increase in dose of medication, it is worth exploring whether there is a specific reason for a worsening of a child's behavior – for example, are they being bullied in school? Are they having academic difficulties? Has their teacher or coach been critical?

Can a child "outgrow" the diagnosis of ADHD?
The diagnosis of ADHD often continues into adulthood. However, the presentation of ADHD can change over time. Hyperactivity often decreases as a child matures; sometimes a child who has been diagnosed with ADHD is diagnosed with alternative mental health diagnoses during

adolescence or adulthood; sometimes their difficulty with organizational skills and focusing continue through adulthood even if they are diagnosed with additional mental health issues. Having a diagnosis of ADHD as a child does increase the risk of adult mental health diagnoses, as well as other social and behavioral issues, including the possibility of "self-medication" with illicit substances or alcohol. However, many children with ADHD do well as adults, learning to compensate for their weaknesses.

Can my child become "addicted" to ADHD medication?

A prescription for stimulant medications typically includes an insert describing potential negative side effects as well as a warning regarding "Abuse and Dependence," stating CNS stimulants have a "high potential for abuse and dependence." However, stimulant medications can be discontinued without the concern for the "withdrawal" symptoms seen in other controlled substance medications (for example, opioids) or illicit substances. Although individuals do not necessarily need to be gradually weaned off a psychostimulant medication, the process of discontinuing medications needs to be managed by the child's treating physician.

Will my child always require treatment with medication?

ADHD can persist into adulthood. Some adults continue to require treatment with medication. However, in the authors' experiences, some children were able to successfully discontinue treatment with medication as early as middle or high school. These individuals require ongoing monitoring for difficulty focusing, as poor focusing can be associated with potential risks (for example, motor vehicle accidents). It is also recommended that individuals with a history of ADHD be monitored for symptoms of alternative mental health diagnoses, as well as monitoring for the risk of "self-medication" with illicit substances, alcohol, etc.

Final note: It is always beneficial to provide your child with ways to comfortably express themself and find positive ways to exude their personality and energy.

BIBLIOGRAPHY

Akinbami, L.J., Liu, X., Pastor, P. N., & Reuben, C.A. (2011). Attention deficit hyperactivity disorder among children ages 5–17 in the United States, 1998–2009. *NICHS Data Brief*, (70).

American Psychiatric Association (APA) (2013). *Diagnostic and Statistical Manual of Mental Disorders – 5th edition*. Arlington, VA: American Psychiatric Association Publishing.

Arnett, A. B., Harsted, E., O'Connell, M., Hayes, K., Brewster, S., Barbaresis, W., & Doan, R. N. (2023). Rare de novo and inherited genes in familial and nonfamilial pediatric attention-deficit/hyperactivity disorder. *Journal of the American Medical Association (JAMA) – Pediatrics*, 178(1): 81–84. https://doi.org/10.1001/jamapediatrics.2023.4952.

Baggio, S., Hasler, R., Glacomini, V., El-Masre, H., Weibel, S., Oerroud, N., & Deiber, M-P. (2019). Does the continuous performance test predict ADHD symptoms severity and ADHD presentation in adults? *Journal of Attention Disorders*, 24(6): 840–848. doi: 10.1177/1087054718822060. Epub 2019 Jan 17.

Barbaresi, W. J., Colligan, R. C., Weaver, A. L., Voigt, R. G., Killian, J. M., Katusic, S. K. (2013). Mortality, ADHD, and psychosocial adversity in adults with childhood ADHD: A prospective study. *Pediatrics*, 131(4), 637–644. doi: 10.1542/peds.2012-2354.

Barbaresi, W. J., Campbell, L, Diekroger, E. A., Froehlich, T. E., Liu, Y. H., O'Malley, E., Pelham, W. E., Power, T. J., Zinner, S. H., & Chan, E. (2020). Society for Developmental and Behavioral Pediatrics clinical practice guideline for the assessment and treatment of children and adolescents with complex attention-deficit/hyperactivity disorder. *Journal of Developmental & Behavioral Pediatrics*, 41 Supplement 2S: S35–S57. doi: 10.1097/DBP.0000000000000770.

Barkley, R. A. (2006). *Attention Deficit Hyperactivity Disorder: A Handbook for Diagnosis and Treatment – 3rd edition*. New York: Guilford Press.

Barkley, R. A. (2015). History of ADHD. In R.A. Barkley (Ed.), *Attention-Deficit Hyperactivity Disorder: A Handbook for Diagnosis and Treatment* (pp. 3–15). New York, NY: The Guilford Press.

Barkley R.A., & Peters, H. (2012). The earliest reference to ADHD in the medical literature? Melchior Adam Weikard's description in 1775 of "attention deficit" (Mangel der Aufmerksmkeit, Attentio Volubilis). *Journal of Attention Disorders*, 16(8): 623–630. https://doi.org/10.1177/1087054711432309. Epub 2012 Feb 8.

Berger, I., Slobodin, O., & Cassuto, H. (2017). Usefulness and validity of continuous performance tests in the diagnosis of attention-deficit hyperactivity disorder children. *Archives of Clinical Neuropsychology*, 32(1): 81–93. https://doi.org/10.1093/arclin/acw101. Epub 2016 Nov 23.

Biederman, J., DiSalvo, M., Vaudreuil, C., Wozniak, J., Uchida, M., Woodworth, K. Y., Green, A., Farrell, A., & Faraone, S. V. (2021). The Child Behavior Checklist can aid in characterizing suspected comorbid psychopathology in clinically referred youth with ADHD. *Journal of Psychiatry Research*, June 138: 477–484. doi: 10.1016/j.jpsychires.2021.04.028. Epub 2021 Apr 30.

Callan, P. D., Eidnes, K., Pope, T. M., Shepler, D. K., Swanberg, S. M., Weber, S. K. (2023). B-46 Diagnostic utility of Conners CPT-3 for ADHD: A systematic review. *Archives of Clinical Neuropsychology*, 38(7): 1410. https://doi.org/10.1093/arclin/acad067.252.

Callan, P. D., Swanberg, S., Weber, S. K., Eines, J., Pope T. M., & Shepler, D. (2024). Diagnostic utility of Conners Continuous Performance Test-3 for attention deficit/hyperactivity disorder: A systematic review. *Journal of Attention Disorders*, 28(6): 992–1007. https://doi.org/10.1177/10870547231223727. Epub 2024 Feb 5.

Chacko, A., Bedard, A. C., Marks, D. J., Feirsen, N., Uderman, J. Z., Chimiklis, A., Rajwan, E., Cornwell, M., Anderson, L., Zwilling, A., & Ramon, M. (2014). A randomized clinical trial of Cogmed working memory training in school-age children with ADHD: A replication in a diverse sample using a control condition. *Journal of Child Psychology and Psychiatry*, 55(3): 247–255. https://doi.org/10.1111/jcpp.12146. Epub 2013 Oct 7.

Children and Adults with Attention-Deficit/Hyperactivity Disorder (CHADD). www.chadd.org.

Chuang, S., & Cooper, T. (2006). Efficacy and safety of immediate-release methylphenidate treatment for preschoolers with ADHD. *Journal of the American Academy of Child and Adolescent Psychiatry*, 45(11): 1284–1293. https://doi.org/10.1097/01.chi.0000235077.32661.61.

Conners, C. K. (2008). *Conners Comprehensive Behavior Rating Scales Manual*. Ontario, Canada: Multi-Health Systems.

Cortese, S., Ferrin, M., Brandeis, D., Buitelaar, J., Daley, D., Dittmann, R. W., Holtmann, M., Santosh, P., Stevenson, J., Stringaris, A., Zuddas, A., Sonuga-Barke, E. J. S., European ADHD Guidelines Group (AGG) (2014). Cognitive training for attention-deficit/hyperactivity disorder: Meta-analysis of clinical and neuropsychological outcomes from randomized controlled trials. *Journal of the American Academy of Child & Adolescent Psychiatry*, 54(3): 164–174. https://doi.org/10.1016/j.jaac.2014.12.010. Epub 2014 Dec 29.

Demontis, D., Lescai, F., Borglum, A., Gierup, S., Ostergarrd, S. D., Mors, O., Li, Q., Liang, J., Jiang, H., Li, Y., Wang, J., Lesch, K-P., Reif, A., Buitelaar, J. K., & Franke, B. (2016). Whole-exome sequencing reveals increased burden of rare functional and disruptive variants in candidate risk genes in individuals with persistent attention-deficit/hyperactivity disorder. *Journal of Academy of Child and Adolescent Psychiatry*, 55(6): 521–523. https://doi.org/10.1016/j.jaac.2016.03.009.

Emser, T. S., Johnston, M. A., Steele, J. D., Kooij, S., Thorell, L., & Christiansen, H. (2018). Assessing ADHD symptoms in children and adults: Evaluating the role of objective measures. *Behavior and Brain Functions*, 14(1): 11. https://doi.org/10.1186/s12993-018-0143-x.

Evans, S. W., Langberg, J. M., Egan, T., Molitor, S. J. (2014). Middle school-based and high school-based interventions for adolescents with ADHD. *Child and Adolescent Psychiatry Clinics of North America*, 23(4): 699–715. https://doi.org/10.1016/j.chc.2014.05.004.

Evans, S. W., Owens, J. S., Wymbs, B. T., Ray, A. R. (2018). Evidence-based psychosocial treatments for children and adolescents with attention deficit/hyperactivity disorder. *Journal of Clinical Child and Adolescent Psychology*, 47(2): 157–198. https://doi.org/10.1080/15374416.2017.1390757. Epub 2017 Dec 19.

Greenberg, L. M., & Waldmant, I. D. (1993). Developmental normative data on the Test of Variables of Attention (T.O.V.A.). *Journal of Child Psychology and Psychiatry*, 24(6): 1019–1030. https://doi.org/10.1111/j.1469-7610.1993.tb01105.x.

Gualtieri, C. T., & Johnson, L. G. (2005) ADHD: Is objective diagnosis possible? *Psychiatry*, 2(11): 44–53.

Hall, C. L., Valentine, A. Z., Walker, G. M., Ball, H. M., Cogger, H., Daley, D., Groom, M. J., Sayal, K., & Hollis, C. (2017). Study of user experience of an objective test (QbTest) to aid ADHD assessment and medication management: A multi-methods approach. *BMC Psychiatry*, 17(1): 66. https://doi.org/10.1186/s12888-017-1222-5.

Harstad, E. B., Katusic, S., Sideridis, G., Weaver, A. L., Voight, R. G., Barbaresis, W. J. (2022). Children with ADHD are at risk for a broad array of adverse adult outcomes that cross functional domains: Results from a population-based birth cohort study. *Journal of Attention Disorders*, 26(1): 3–14. https://doi.org/10.1177/1087054720964578. Epub 2020 Oct 22.

Hennissen, L., Bakker, M. J., Banaschewski, T., Carucci, S., Coghill, D., Danckaerts, M., Dittman, R. W., Hollis, C., Kovshoff, H., McCarthy, S., Nagy, P., Sonuga-Barke, E., Wong, I. C. K., Zuddas, A., Rosenthal, E., Buitlaar, J. K., ADDUCE Consortium (2017). Cardiovascular effects of stimulant and non-stimulant medication for children and adolescents with ADHD: A systematic review and meta-analysis of trials of methylphenidate, amphetamines and atomoxetine. *CNS Drugs*, 31(3): 199–215. https://doi.org/10.1007/s40263-017-0410-7.

Hollis, C., Falconer, C. J., Martin, J. L., Whittington, C., Stockton, S., Glazebrook, C., & Davies, E. B. (2017). Annual research review: Digital health interventions for children and young people with mental health problems—A systematic and meta-review. *Journal of Child Psychology and Psychiatry*, 58(4): 474–503. https://doi.org/10.1111/jcpp.12663. Epub 2016 Dec 10.

Jarratt K. P., Riccio C. A., & Siekierski B. M. (2005). Assessment of attention deficit hyperactivity disorder (ADHD) using the BASC and BRIEF. *Applied Neuropsychology*, 12(2): 83–93. https://doi.org/10.1207/s15324826an1202_4.

Jensen P. S., Hinshaw, S. P., Swanson, J. M., Greenhill, L. L., Conners, C. K., Arnold, L. E., Abikoff, H. B., Elliott, G., Hechtman, L., Hoza, B., March, J. S., Newcorn, J. H., Severe, J. B., Vitiello, B., Wells, K., & Wigal, T. (2002). Findings from the NIMH Multimodal Treatment Study of ADHD (MTA): Implications and applications for primary care providers. *Journal of Developmental and Behavioral Pediatrics*, 22(1): 60–73. https://doi.org/10.1097/00004703-200102000-00008.

Klein, R. G., Mannuzza, S., Olazagasti, M. A., Roizen, E., Hutchison, J. A., Lashua, E. C., & Castellanos, F. X. (2012). Clinical and functional outcome of childhood attention-deficit/hyperactivity disorder 33 years later. *Archives of General Psychiatry*, 69(12), 1295–1303. https://doi.org/10.1001/archgenpsychiatry.2012.271.

Kollins, S. H., DeLoss, D. J., Canadas, E., Lutz, J., Findling, R. L., Keefe, S. E., Epstein, J. N., Cutler, A. J., & Faraone, S. V. (2020). A novel digital intervention for actively reducing severity of paediatric ADHD (STARS-ADHD): A randomised controlled trial. *Lancet Digital Health*, 2(4): e168–e178. https://doi.org/10.1016/S2589-7500(20)30017-0. Epub 2020 Feb 24.

Lee, S. S., Humphreys, K. L., Flory, K., Liu, R., & Glass, K. (2011). Prospective association of childhood attention-deficit/hyperactivity disorder (ADHD) and substance use and abuse/dependence: A meta-analytic review. *Clinical Psychology Review*, 31(3), 328–341. https://doi.org/10.1016/j.cpr.2011.01.006. Epub 2011 Jan 20.

Levy, S., Katusic, S. K., Colligan, R. C., Weaver, A. L., Killian, J. M., Voigt, R. G., Barbaresi, W. J. (2014). Childhood ADHD and risk for substance dependence in adulthood: A longitudinal, population-based study. *PLoS One*, 9(8), e105640. https://doi.org/10.1371/journal.pone.0105640.

McGough, J. J., Sturm, A., Cowen, J., Tung, K., Salgari, G. C., Leuchte, A.F., Cook, I. A., Sugar, C. A., & Loo, S. K. (2019). Double-blind, sham-controlled, pilot study of trigeminal nerve stimulation for attention-deficit/hyperactivity disorder. *Journal of the American Academy of Child and Adolescent Psychiatry*, 58(4): 403–411.e3. https://doi.org/10.1016/j.jaac.2018.11.013. Epub 2019 Jan 28.

Mick, E., McManus, D. D., & Goldberg, R. J. (2013). Meta-analysis of increased heart rate and blood pressure associated with CNS stimulant treatment of ADHD in adults. *European Neuropsychopharmacology*, 23(6): 534–541. https://doi.org/10.1016/j.euroneuro.2012.06.011. Epub 2012 Jul 15.

Morrison, J. (2014) *DSM-5 Made Easy. The Clinician's Guide to Diagnosis.* New York, NY: The Guilford Press.

The MTA Cooperative Group (1999). Multimodal Treatment Study of Children with ADHD. A 14-month randomized clinical trial of treatment strategies for attention-deficit/hyperactivity disorder. *Archives of General Psychiatry*, 56(12): 1073–1086. https://doi.org/10.1001/archpsyc.56.12.1073.

National Institute for Children's Health Quality (2002). *NICHQ Vanderbilt Assessment Scale.* Elk Grove Village, IL: American Academy of Pediatrics. McNeill Consumer and Specialty Pharmaceuticals.

Norman, L.J., Sudre, G., Price, J., & Shaw, P. L. (2024). Subcortico-cortical dysconnectivity in ADHD. A voxel-wise mega-analysis across multiple cohorts. *American Journal of Psychiatry*. https://ajp.psychiatryonline.org/doi/10.1176/appi.ajp.20230026.

Office of the Assistant Secretary for Administration and Management, US Dept of Labor (1973). *Section 504, Rehabilitation Act.* Washington, D.C.: US Department of Health and Human Services.

Oldrati, V., Corti, C., Poggi, G., Borgatti, R., Uresi, C., & Bardoni, A. (2020). Effectiveness of computerized cognitive training programs (CCTP) with game-like features in children with or without neuropsychological disorders: A meta-analytic investigation. *Neuropsychology Review*, 30(1): 126–141. https://doi.org/10.1007/s11065-020-09429-5. Epub 2020 Feb 28.

Pan, X.-X., Ma, H.-W., & Dai, X.-M. (2007). Value of integrated visual and auditory continuous performance test in the diagnosis of childhood attention deficit hyperactivity disorder (article in Chinese). *Zhongguo Dang Dai Er Ke Za Zhi*, 9(3): 210–220.

Peterson, B. S., Trampush, J., Brown, J., Maglione, M., Bolshakova, M., Rozelle, M., Miles, J., Pakdaman, S., Brown, M., Yagyu, S., Motala, A., & Hempel, S. (2024a). Treatments for ADHD in children and adolescents: A systematic review. *Pediatrics*, e2024065787. https://doi.org/10.1542/peds.2024-065787.

Peterson, B. S., Trampush, J., Brown, M., Maglione, M., Bolshakova, M., Rozelle, M., Miles, J., Pakdaman, S., Yagyu, S., Motala, A., & Hempel, S.

(2024b). Tools for the diagnosis of ADHD in children and adolescents: A systematic review. *Pediatrics*, e2024065854. https://doi.org/10.1542/peds.2024-065854.

Reuben, C., & Elgaddal, M. S. (2024). Attention-deficit/hyperactivity disorder in children ages 5–17 years: United States, 2020–2022. *National Center for Health Statistics Data Brief*, (499): 1–9.

Roebuk, H., Freigang, C., & Barry, J. G. (2016) Continuous performance tasks: Not just about sustaining attention. *Journal of Speech, Language, and Hearing Research*, 59(3): 501–510. doi: 10.1044/2015_JSLHR-L-15-0068.

Shaked, D., Faulkner, L. M. D., Tolle, K., Wendell, C. R., Waldstein, S. R., & Spencer, R. J. (2020). Reliability and validity of the Conners' Continuous Performance Test. *Applied Neuropsychology Adult*, 27(5): 478–487. https://doi.org/10.1080/23279095.2019.1570199. Epub 2019 Feb 22. https://doi.org/10.1080/23279095.2019.1598087.

Shepard, S. A., & Dickstein, S. (2009). Preventive intervention for early childhood behavioral problems: An ecological perspective. *Child and Adolescent Psychiatry Clinics of North America*, 18(3): 687–706. https://doi.org/10.1016/j.chc.2009.03.002.

Smith, M. (2012). *Hyperactive: The Controversial History of ADHD*. London, England: Reaktion Books.

Thapar, A. (2018). Discoveries on the genetics of ADHD in the 21st century: New findings and their implications. *The American Journal of Psychiatry*, 175: 943–950. https://doi.org/10.1176/appi.ajp.2018.18040383. Epub 2018 Aug 16,

Tinius, T. P. (2003). The Integrated Visual and Auditory Continuous Performance Test as a neuropsychological measure. *Archives of Clinical Neuropsychology*, 18(5): 439–454. https://doi.org/10.1016/S0887-6177(02)00144-0.

Understood.org. www.understood.org.

Webster-Stratton, C. H., Reid, M. J., & Beauchaine, T. (2011). Combining parent and child training for young children with ADHD. *Journal of Clinical Child and Adolescent Psychology*, 40(2): 191–203. https://doi.org/10.1080/15374416.2011.546044.

Wilens, T. E., Carrellas, N. W., Zulauf, C., Yule, A. M., Uchida, M., Spencer, A., & Biederman, J. (2017). Pilot data supporting omega-3 fatty acids supplementation in medicated children with attention-deficit/hyperactivity disorder and deficits in emotional self-regulation. *Journal of Child and Adolescent Psychopharmacology*, 27(8): 755–756. https://doi.org/10.1089/cap.2017.0080. Epub 2017 Jun 29.

Wolraich, M. L., Hagan, J. F., Allan, C., Chan, E., Davison, D., Earls, M., Evans, S. W., Flinn, S. K., Froehlich, T., Frost, J., Holbrook, J. R., Lehmann, C. U., Lessin, H. R., Okechukwau, K., Pierce, K. L.,

Winner, J. D., & Zuhellen, W. (Subcommittee on Children and Adolescents with Attention-Deficit/Hyperative Disorder) (2019). Clinical practice guideline for the diagnosis, evaluation, and treatment of attention-deficit/hyperactivity disorder in children and adolescents. *Pediatrics*, 144(4): e20192528. https://doi.org/10.1542/peds.2019-3997.

Xu, G., Strathearn, L., Liu, B., Yang, M., & Bao, W. (2018) Twenty-year trends in diagnosed attention-deficit/hyperactivity disorder among US children and adolescents, 1997–2016. *Journal of the American Medical Association*. 1(4): e181471. https://doi.org/10.1001/jamanetworkopen.2018.1471.

Zhang, L., Li, L., Andell, P., Garcia-Argibay, M., Quinn, P. D., D'Onofrio, B. M., Brikell, I., Kuja-Halkola, R., Lichtenstein, P., Johnell, K., Larsson, H., & Change, Z. (2024) Attention-deficit/hyperactivity disorder medications and long-term risk of cardiovascular diseases. *Journal of the American Medical Association Psychiatry*, 81(2): 178–187. https://doi.org/10.1001/jamapsychiatry.2023.4294.

Zhang, L., Yao, H., Li, L., Rietz, E. D., Andell, P., Garcia-Argibay, M., D'Onofrio, B. M., Coreses, S., Larsson, H., & Chang, Z. (2022). Risk of cardiovascular diseases associated with medications used in attention-deficit/hyperactivity disorder. A systematic review and meta-analysis. *Journal of the American Medical Association Open*, 5(11): e2243597. https://doi.org/10.1001/jamanetworkopen.2022.43597.

CHAPTER 6

Oppositional Defiant Disorder or Just Strong Willed?

Let us begin this chapter with a brief discussion regarding the skepticism that has existed toward some mental health diagnoses, particularly behaviorally-based disorders. A parent once told me that if her child had a physical disability, other people would be empathetic and offer support, but because her child had a behavioral disorder, people gave her "looks", suggesting that she must be a poor parent.

In actuality, no individual, child or adult, demonstrates what others consider acceptable behavior 100% of the time. Moreover, tantrums and oppositionality are part of typical child development. Learning what is considered an acceptable behavior and learning to regulate and manage behavior and emotions are part of a child's journey to maturity and independence. A child's impulsive behavior may be due to them not yet having acquired the skill of being able to "think before acting." Children are each "wired" differently and present with their own unique disposition, which can sometimes be reflected in their behavior.

In addition to a child's developmental level, personality, and inherent character qualities, a child's behavior can also be considered a way for a child to communicate – a child's negative behavior may be their way of letting you know that they are feeling angry, sad, or anxious; or maybe they are in need of some extra attention.

So, if behavioral challenges are part of typical growth and development, why do we provide a mental health diagnosis for some children who demonstrate behavioral challenges? Sometimes a child's negative behaviors are much more extreme than what is considered typical for their age. Their unacceptable behaviors cannot be explained simply by their strong-willed personality and have a negative impact on their functioning at home, school, and in the community, as well as a negative impact on family functioning. Similar to diagnoses discussed in previous chapters (i.e., intellectual

DOI: 10.4324/9781003639121-6

disability [ID], autism spectrum disorder [ASD], and attention-deficit/hyperactivity disorder [ADHD]), one can think of a "bell shaped curve" of behaviors in children, with a "spectrum" of presentations. Behavioral issues at the lower end of the curve or spectrum regarding their degree of maladaptive behaviors and their intensity and frequency may be considered outside the range of typical childhood behavior, and may meet criteria for a behavioral disorder. More specifically, the chapter will discuss whether the intensity and frequency of a child's angry and irritable mood and oppositional and negative behaviors may meet criteria for the diagnosis of oppositional defiant disorder (ODD). The validity of ODD as a unique mental health disorder has been studied extensively and has been supported in many research studies (Aggarwal & Marwaha, 2022; Burke et al., 2022; Greene et al., 2002; Hudziak et al., 2005; Keenan & Shaw, 2003; Rey et al., 1988; Rutter et al., 1998).

CASE STUDIES

Elijah is two-and-a-half years old, and he has been saying "no" in response to almost all requests. When he is told "no", this can result in him kicking and screaming for sometimes as long as five minutes. Elijah's parents are frustrated with his behavior, and their neighbor told them that he may have ODD.

Luna's first grade teacher reported that Luna has not been compliant with completing her school work – she often places her head down on her desk and does not respond to her teacher's requests. At home she has always enjoyed playing with toys. She has not always been responsive to instructions, but her behavior has never been considered problematic. Luna's teacher questioned whether Luna's parents were not disciplining her appropriately at home or whether there were some family issues that Luna has been experiencing. The teacher also suggested that maybe Luna should be evaluated to assess for behavioral diagnoses such as ODD.

Aiden was just suspended from kindergarten and had previously been asked to leave three different preschools because of his unacceptable behavior. He had difficulty sharing and could demonstrate severe tantrums in response to the word, "no." His tantrums sometimes resulted in the other children in his class needing to leave the room for their own safety. At home Aiden gets into frequent fights with his siblings. His parents reported that it makes them sad to see him always appear so irritable and often unhappy. Aiden's parents read about the diagnosis of ODD and asked your opinion about this diagnosis.

OPPOSITIONAL DEFIANT DISORDER (ODD)

Oppositional defiant disorder is a type of behavioral disorder. A child with this diagnosis can present with many behavioral features that are commonly seen in childhood. However, with the diagnosis of ODD, these behaviors are observed to be more intense, persistent, and problematic than what is considered appropriate for the child's age. Oppositional defiant disorder can be described as mild, moderate, or severe, depending on the number of settings in which a child exhibits their negative behaviors. If the behaviors are observed in only one setting, it is considered "mild"; in two settings, it is considered "moderate"; and in three or more settings, it is considered "severe" (American Psychiatric Association [APA], 2013; Morrison, 2014). In order to make this diagnosis, a thorough history and exam are needed, and other diagnoses should be considered.

AUTHORS' COMMENTARY

Although negative behaviors can be a characteristic of typical child development, the diagnosis of ODD has "stood the test of time" as a valid mental health diagnosis. Although there are risks to "over-medicalizing" children's behavior, a specific diagnosis can often enable a child and their family to access services to address challenging behaviors. In a recent article, Scott refuted the idea that providing a diagnosis of a behavioral disorder, including ODD, during childhood can have a negative impact on the child and/or family. He also discussed the importance of treating specific negative behaviors appropriately, regardless of the specific diagnosis (Scott, 2022). Burke and colleagues also refuted the idea that ODD is a medicalization of normative childhood behavior, a reflection only of social and family issues, or just a form or symptoms of alternative mental health diagnoses (Burke et al., 2022).

DIAGNOSING ODD

As with all diagnoses, it is important to obtain a detailed child and family history as part of an evaluation for ODD. Is the family situation stable? Has the child experienced trauma? Have they been the victim of bullying? Is there a strong family history of individuals with mental health diagnoses? Is the child's behavior more suggestive of other developmental or mental health diagnoses – for example, ADHD, anxiety, depression, or ASD?

It is important to obtain information from multiple informants, including parents/guardians, siblings, teachers, school counselors, etc. Results of cognitive and academic testing are also beneficial. Similar to ADHD, there are several surveys and questionnaires that can be used to help make a definitive diagnosis of ODD, some of which listed alphabetically below.

Behavior Assessment System for Children 2nd edition (BASC-2) and the BASC-2 Behavioral and Emotional Screening System (BASC-2 BESS)

These are designed to assess the behavioral and emotional strengths and weaknesses of children aged 3–18 years old. Components include a teacher rating scale, a parent rating scale, and a self-report of personality. The results can provide information for an assessment for behavioral and emotional disorders in children (Kamphaus & Reynolds, 2007).

The Child and Adolescent Psychiatric Assessment

This is an interview-based evaluation of symptoms and severity ratings for mental health diagnoses in children and adolescents aged 9–17 years old (Angold & Costello, 2000).

Child Behavior Checklist (CBCL)

This is a well-known caregiver report survey used to identify behavioral problems in children. It is a component of the **Achenbach System of Empirically Based Assessment** developed by Thomas M. Achenbach (Achenbach & Rescorla, 2001). Of note, Biederman and colleagues evaluated the clinical scales of the CBCL in children with ADHD and found that the CBCL Aggression Scale was predictive of ODD behaviors (Biederman et al., 2008).

Conduct and Oppositional Defiant Disorder Scales (CODDS)

This is a 23 item caregiver and self-report evaluation tool based on the *Diagnostic and Statistical Manual of Mental Disorders – 5th edition* (DSM-5) (APA, 2013) criteria for both ODD and conduct disorder. In a 2022 article, Raine and colleagues reported on two studies assessing the validity and reliability of this screening tool. Results revealed that the CODDS has good sensitivity and specificity in predicting the diagnoses of ODD and CD (Raine et al., 2022).

Conners' Rating Scales

Although the Conners' Scale is typically associated with an evaluation for the diagnosis of ADHD, the scale includes an oppositional subscale. Kuny and colleagues utilized a multilevel latent class analysis of Conners' Parent Scale Oppositional subscale with comparisons made to maternal CBCL scores. The results enabled them to differentiate symptoms into several classes of ODD behaviors (Kuny et al., 2013).

Development and Well-Being Assessment (DAWBA)

This includes questionnaires, interviews, and rating scales designed to assess for psychiatric diagnoses in children and adolescents aged 5–16 years old (Goodman et al., 2000).

National Institute of Mental Health Diagnostic Interview Schedule for Children (NIMH DISC-IV)

This is a structured, computer-based diagnostic instrument that was designed to assess for psychiatric disorders in children based on DSM criteria (Shaffer et al., 2000). The tool includes modules that can be used to assess for ODD (Shaffer et al., 2000; Raine et al., 2022).

Oppositional Defiant Disorder Rating Scale (ODDRS)

This scale is designed to assess for symptoms of ODD. A 2010 study by O'Laughlin and colleagues found that children who had been diagnosed with ODD based on parent interviews had elevated scores on the parent version of the ODDRS compared to those who had not been diagnosed with ODD. Classification ratings for the ODDRS were similar to classification ratings based on the aggression subscale of the BASC-2. Of note, the Teacher ratings did not discriminate between the ODD and non-ODD groups (O'Laughlin et al., 2010).

Strength and Difficulties Questionnaire (SDQ)

This is a questionnaire used to screen for behavioral and emotional symptoms in children and adolescents (Grasso et al., 2022).

PREVALENCE OF ODD

Reports of ODD prevalence are variable, ranging from 1% to 16% (Aggarwal & Marwaha, 2022; Nock et al., 2007). This large range is possibly related to different informant sources, retrospective vs. current data, and whether some prevalence data regarding ODD also include the diagnosis of conduct disorder. There are more males than females diagnosed with ODD during childhood/preadolescence (Aggarwal & Marwaha, 2022), and a diagnosis of ODD is associated with an increased risk of other mental health diagnoses, both concurrently and in the future (Aggarwal & Marwaha, 2022; Nock, et al., 2007).

It has been reported that children in racial minorities are more likely to be diagnosed with ODD, with racism considered a possible contributing factor to over-diagnosing (Legha, 2025). Legha recently proposed an "antiracist" approach to considering this diagnosis, which includes recognition of society's potential racial biases and focusing on a child's psychosocial history, possible other mental health challenges, and avoiding describing challenging behaviors as "features of the child" and more an expression of their neurodevelopmental profile (Legha, 2025).

WHAT CAUSES ODD?

The etiology of ODD is felt to likely be multifactorial, with possible genetic, psychological, social, and environmental contributing factors (Aggarwal & Marwaha, 2022; Riley et al., 2016). As with many other mental health diagnoses, a family history of ODD increases a child's risk for this disorder, as well as other behaviorally-based diagnoses. Prenatal risk factors (for example, nicotine and illicit substance exposure, nutritional deficiencies) can increase a child's risk for multiple challenges, including behavioral problems associated with ODD (Riley et al., 2016). Moreover, high-risk environments, such as poverty, parental mental health diagnoses, and community violence, are risk factors for several mental health disorders, including ODD. There have also been studies exploring the possible biological/neurological contributions of neurotransmitters and cortisol levels, and neuroimaging findings associated with this diagnosis (Aggarwal & Marwaha, 2022).

OTHER BEHAVIORAL DISORDERS CAN SHARE BEHAVIORS WITH ODD AND CAN ALSO OCCUR CO-MORBIDLY WITH ODD

Behaviors associated with ODD can also be observed in children with alternative diagnoses, including ASD (Chapter 4) and ADHD (Chapter 5). It is also not uncommon for children with ODD to be diagnosed with co-morbid mental health diagnoses. Finally, a child's diagnosis of ODD may transition to an alternative mental health diagnosis in the future. When a child presents with behaviors suggestive of ODD, it is important to explore possible causes for the child's behavior, as well as consider alternative and additional diagnoses. Is this child's behavior associated with anxiety or depression? Is this child's behavior a result of a history of trauma?

Conduct Disorder

Conduct disorder (CD) is a behavioral disorder that is typically considered to be more severe than ODD. Conduct disorder can be associated with school truancy, property damage, stealing, and physical aggression (APA 2013; Morrison, 2014). A relationship between ODD and CD has been suggested, with a percentage of children with ODD later being diagnosed with CD. The two diagnoses have sometimes been grouped together in research studies and some studies have treated them as if they are part of a spectrum of a single diagnosis. However, there is also evidence reported that they are distinct diagnoses (Aggarwal & Marwaha, 2022; APA, 2013; Morrison J, 2014; Hudziak et al., 2005; Rowe et al., 2011).

ADHD

The association between ODD and ADHD is well-studied. ADHD as a single diagnosis can be associated with some behaviors associated with ODD, and should be considered as the primary diagnosis if a child's impulsivity, high activity level, inattention, and/or distractibility appear to be their most significant challenges. However, ADHD and ODD can also be co-morbid diagnoses (Aggarwal & Marwaha, 2022).

Anxiety

Anxiety is reviewed in Chapter 8. Anxiety in children can also present with irritability and behavioral problems and should therefore be considered in children who present with features of ODD. It is possible that an anxiety disorder may be the primary diagnoses or a co-morbid diagnosis.

Mood Disorders

Children with ODD can exhibit irritability, as well as emotional dys-regulation and lability, which can also be characteristics of mood disorders, including depression. It is important to establish if a child's primary diagnosis is a mood disorder before providing them with a definitive diagnosis of ODD. However, similar to ADHD, mood disorders can co-occur with ODD (Aggarwal & Marwaha, 2022). It is notable that ODD is a more common diagnosis than mood disorders in younger children. However, it is important to re-evaluate a child's mental health and presentation over time, assessing for additional and alternative diagnoses as they mature. Some children who were initially diagnosed with ODD, may transition to alternative diagnoses, including mood disorders, later in life.

Disruptive Mood Dysregulation Disorder (DMDD)

DMDD was a diagnosis added to the DSM-5. The diagnosis of DMDD shares features with ODD, but it is not diagnosed in children who are younger than six and includes a more intense and chronic presentation of negative behaviors and irritability in multiple settings. Overall, DMDD is considered a more severe behavioral disorder than ODD (Aggarwal & Marwaha, 2022; APA, 2013).

Impairing Emotional Outbursts

Impairing emotional outbursts is a condition that was added to the DSM-5-TR, published in 2022. It is characterized by episodes of intense outbursts that are much more severe than what would typically be expected for the circumstances. These behavioral/emotional outbursts can occur as part of specific diagnoses such as DMDD or ODD (APA, 2022).

Post-Traumatic Stress Disorder (PTSD)

This diagnosis is discussed in Chapter 11. It is notable that children who experience trauma can present with a variety of behavioral and mood issues associated with the diagnosis of ODD.

AUTHORS' COMMENTARY

Although a diagnosis of ODD can provide a "label" for a child's negative behaviors, this should not result in the behaviors being considered acceptable, i.e., the diagnosis may help "explain" the behaviors but should not be an "excuse" for the behaviors. Regardless of a diagnosis, therapists and other adults in the child's life should attempt to understand any historical context and possible precipitants/triggers for a child's negative behaviors, as well as explore treatments and supports to correct the child's unacceptable behaviors. After it is determined that the most appropriate diagnosis for a child is ODD, intensive behavioral supports need to be explored. In addition, parents should not feel that they are being "blamed" for a child's misbehavior, but they should be part of the process to better understand and modify the behaviors.

FUNCTIONAL BEHAVIORAL ANALYSIS (FBA)

Before discussing treatments and supports for children with ODD, let us take a slight detour and re-explore a Functional Behavioral Analysis (FBA). An FBA, also sometimes referred to as a functional behavioral assessment, was discussed briefly in previous chapters. Since ODD is a behavioral disorder, exploring an FBA in more detail appears appropriate for this chapter. An FBA examines specific behaviors that are interfering with a child's functioning, and can be completed for a child with or without a behavioral diagnosis.

Goals of the assessment, which is often completed at school, include identifying specific factors that precipitate a child's negative behaviors, determining the purpose of the behaviors, and the function/outcome the child gains or attempts to gain by the behavior. After these factors are identified, a plan can be made to address and hopefully correct the negative behaviors (Merlo et al., 2018).

Examples of negative behaviors that could be considered "target behaviors" that are often observed in children with ODD include the following:

- behavior outbursts due to poor emotional regulation and/or limited frustration tolerance;
- immediate argument and/or outburst in response to being refused a preferred activity or item or being requested to perform a nonpreferred activity;
- immediate and persistent negative responses to peers and adults.

Let us describe some possible triggers for negative behaviors:

- academic, behavioral, and/or social demands;
- information "overload";
- being informed they are wrong/incorrect; feeling that they are always being told "no";
- frustration when things do not go as anticipated;
- feeling "always forced" to do what others want them to do;
- feeling they are not believed, listened to, or treated fairly.

Some possible "functions" of the negative behaviors may include:

- reacting to and attempting to eliminate stress or "overload";
- avoiding/escaping demands or expectation;
- reducing/avoiding stress and anxiety of social interactions and demands;
- attempting to manage and avoid overwhelming situations/events/ experiences;
- gaining attention of adults (even if the attention is not positive).

Despite the "function" of these behaviors, it is important to note that there are also typically negative consequences for the child's unacceptable behavior, such as time away from positive experiences and/or continual worsening of the child's self-esteem. Moreover, despite their attempt to decrease their feelings of being overloaded, the child may ultimately feel even more emotionally overloaded and overwhelmed by their behaviors.

Examples of strategies to address some of these target behaviors at school and outside of school include the following:

- increased staff-supported small group interactive activities;
- structured activities with peers/staff that reduce interpersonal/interactive stress/anxiety;
- recognition of the child's social isolation, and attempts to replace it with positive peer socialization experiences;
- rewards/incentives/reinforcements provided when expected/appropriate behaviors occur;
- allotted time/number of reinforcements increased as frequencies of areas of concern decrease;
- self-calming strategies (for example, self-relaxation, self-soothing) and other stress management techniques;
- creation of an incentive chart;

- increased time with preferred activities as reward for appropriate behavior;
- time with preferred adults;
- generation of additional replacement and preference behaviors and opportunities for positive reinforcement.

Let us now return to Elijah, Luna, and Aiden.

CASE STUDIES

Elijah's pediatrician felt that Elijah's tantrums were appropriate for his age and also felt that two-and-a-half years old was too young to make a definitive diagnosis of ODD. Elijah's parents were instructed to place Elijah in a safe place during his tantrums and attempt to ignore the behavior. Other behavioral strategies were also discussed. Instead of asking questions that could result in Elijah responding "no!", Elijah's parents began giving him choices – for example, instead of saying, "It's dinner time, come to the table," they asked, "Would you rather sit in the end seat for dinner or between Daddy and Mommy?" Elijah's tantrums gradually decreased over time and his compliance gradually improved. Elijah also began attending a play group and enjoyed spending time with peers.

Luna had a multidisciplinary team evaluation completed by the public school system. Results of speech-language testing revealed variable scores. There were some mild delays in Luna's expressive language and some of her receptive language scores were even more significantly impaired. There were concerns regarding Luna's ability to understand and process information (her parents were informed that she was too young to have a central auditory processing evaluation completed). A full audiology assessment was completed, and Luna was diagnosed with unilateral hearing loss. An individualized education program (IEP) was created which included speech-language therapy and classroom supports and accommodations.

Aiden also had a multidisciplinary team evaluation completed by the public school system and his language and early learning skills were both reported to be within the average range. A functional behavior analysis was completed, and an intensive behavioral plan was created. Aiden also had additional psychological testing completed outside of school and was diagnosed with severe ODD, as his negative behaviors had been observed at home, at school, and also in public places and relatives' homes. Although Aiden's parents were informed that Aiden's diagnosis of ODD did not necessarily qualify him for an IEP, the special education team felt that Aiden's behavioral challenges were extensive enough for an IEP to be created in order to maximize the behavioral supports he would be able to receive at school.

THERAPIES AND INTERVENTIONS FOR CHILDREN WITH ODD

A treatment plan for a child with ODD optimally involves a team approach, including the child and their parents/guardians and possibly other family members, teachers, school counselor and school behavioral support team, and community resources, including a therapist/counselor. A detailed family, social, and school history should be obtained, to identify a family history of mental health challenges, peer relationship issues, learning challenges, and other health issues.

Additional diagnoses, such ADHD and mood disorders, should also be explored, as this may modify the treatment plan. Finally, assessment of a child's interpersonal attachments, their relationship with their parents and siblings, and the parents' beliefs regarding appropriate methods of raising a child add important information in order to explore optimal treatment approaches (Aggarwal & Marwaha, 2022).

Evidenced-based treatments for children with ODD include family-based interventions such as parent management training, school supports, and individual treatment such as behavioral counseling/therapy. Parenting techniques such as providing structure and consistency and positively rewarding appropriate behavior can be challenging for a child who is very oppositional. Therefore, working with a mental health professional is of primary importance when providing treatment for children with ODD. With preschool children, the first line of therapy is typically parent education and training, with play therapy sometimes incorporated into the program. For school-age children, a combination of school-based interventions, family-based treatment, and individual therapy can be included into the program. In adolescents, individual therapy is often implemented in combination with school and family supports and services (Aggarwal & Marwaha, 2022).

Parent Management Training

Working with a mental health consultant/counselor/therapist to develop parental skills to improve a child's behavior can decrease family stress (Wise, 2022). Parent management training teaches the implementation of positive reinforcement to decrease unacceptable behaviors and facilitate appropriate behavior (Aggarwal & Marwaha, 2022; Kazdin et al., 2018). There have been multiple randomized controlled trials, the results of which support parent training. The programs assist parents in learning techniques to facilitate improvements in their child's behavioral and emotional regulation, and teaches them positive reinforcement techniques and how to provide appropriate consequences for negative behavior (Leijten et al., 2022). Follow up studies have revealed lasting benefits from these programs (Scott et al., 2014). Of note, **parent–child interaction therapy** is a behaviorally based type of Parent Management Training that implements play-based interaction techniques in addition to behaviorally based techniques (Funderbunk & Eyberg, 2011).

Family Therapy

Living with a child who demonstrates behavioral challenges can be stressful for other family members. Family therapy may be beneficial as a supplemental therapy. In addition to exploring ways to decrease family stress, the therapist can work with family members to explore possible triggers to the child's maladaptive behaviors and also explore additional inter-personal dynamics among family members.

Individual Therapy

Individual therapy for children with ODD should be geared to the child's age and specific challenging behaviors.

Cognitive Behavioral Therapy (CBT)

This therapy teaches coping strategies and desensitization strategies to change negative behaviors and improve behavioral regulation. CBT was mentioned in previous chapters and will be discussed further in future chapters. Implementing CBT-based anger-management training can be useful in treating a child or adolescent with anger issues. In addition, problem-solving and perspective-taking training are CBT tools that can be beneficial to older children and adolescents who demonstrate aggressive types of behaviors (Lochman et al., 2011).

Play Therapy

This therapy involves a therapist/counselor working with a child through play to explore the child's behavioral response to various situations. It teaches them acceptable and positive ways to deal with situations that previously resulted in negative behaviors (Jafari et al., 2011).

School-based Interventions and Supports

A school-based behavioral plan is important for children with ODD. Some children qualify for an IEP, typically if they have learning challenges in addition to their behavioral disorder. However, in our experience, if a child who is diagnosed with a behavioral disorder only demonstrates behaviors that result in their inability to function in school and/or is considered a safety risk to themselves or others, the school may still determine that an IEP is needed. If a child's behavior disorder does not qualify them for an IEP, then creation of a 504 Accommodation Plan would be appropriate if there are behavioral problems observed at school. Many teachers have a general behavioral plan in their classroom. However, a child with ODD may require an individual school behavioral plan to target their specific behavioral problems and improve their emotional and behavioral regulation, peer relations, and problem-solving skills.

Medication

Behavioral interventions, therapies, and supports are the primary treatments for symptoms of ODD. Although there are no medications designed specifically to treat ODD, sometimes a trial of treatment with medication may be initiated to treat co-morbid diagnoses – for example, ADHD, depression, or anxiety. In addition, if a child with a behavioral disorder continues to present with severe behavioral challenges (for example, that pose a safety risk, despite maximum supports and behavioral interventions) a consulting psychiatrist may feel that a trial of treatment with medication is indicated to explore whether medication will result in an improvement in the child's functioning and quality of life.

As discussed in Chapter 5, treatment with psychostimulant medication is typically the first line of medication treatment for ADHD. Although many children with ODD and ADHD can be successfully treated with stimulant medication, some children with ODD may experience negative side effects such as irritability or emotional lability, and may benefit more from a non-stimulant medication. For example, guanfacine sometimes helps decrease impulsivity and can have a calming effect, i.e., it "takes the edge off", for a child with ODD. The medication, Risperidone, was discussed in Chapter 4, as it has been approved for treatment of children with ASD who demonstrate severe dysregulation and/or aggression. Risperidone and some of the other medications classified as "atypical antipsychotics" are sometimes used to treat aggressive behaviors in children with behavioral disorders. It should be noted, however, that these medications (as well as medications in the category of "mood stabilizers," which include some antiepileptic medications) have risks of negative side effects and should therefore be used with caution and typically under the supervision of a child psychiatrist.

CASE STUDIES

When **Elijah** was three years old, he began attending a structured inclusion preschool program as a community student. He responded positively to a behavioral plan at school and proudly informed his parents each time he received a positive behavioral report from his teachers. Elijah had a fairly successful school experience through high school, with only occasional challenges that were considered age-appropriate, and similar to his peers.

It was not felt that **Luna** required a hearing aid, but she continued to qualify for an IEP during elementary school based on her diagnosis of unilateral hearing deficit and a communication disorder. When Luna was eight years old, she was also diagnosed with an auditory processing disorder – this is considered a learning disability, and her unilateral hearing deficit was not felt to be the direct cause of this diagnosis. Luna required less support over time, and her IEP was discontinued prior to her senior year of high school. She attended college and earned a degree in website design.

Aiden continued to work with a therapist outside of school and also received in-school counseling. Although his behavior continued to be challenging, he was able to function in a kindergarten classroom that provided him with intensive supports.

Aiden's parents continued to work with his therapist on strategies to learn to better manage Aiden's behavior. However, Aiden's school journey was not easy. During elementary school it was questioned whether some of his behaviors may be related to a diagnosis of ADHD, and a trial of treatment with medication was initiated. Initially some mild improvement in Aiden's impulsivity was observed, associated with treatment with medication, but the efficacy of the medication decreased over time. After multiple trials of different medications, it was decided to give Aiden a "break" from medication. In fifth grade, Aiden was reported to lie to adults and was also caught stealing from a store. A diagnosis of CD was then considered by his therapist. Aiden transitioned into a therapeutic public-school program designed for students with behavioral challenges. The program included intensive behavioral and social-emotional supports. Aiden continued to receive individual therapy, and his family received family therapy outside of school. A gradual improvement in Aiden's behavior was observed.

Aiden's family and the staff at school were pleasantly surprised during middle school, during which time Aiden continued to participate in an intensive behaviorally based program but was able to function fairly well. He did not receive any suspensions from school during eigth grade. Aiden successfully attended a vocational program in high school, and he continued to be closely monitored by a counselor and psychiatrist for mental health diagnoses and risk for substance use. Aiden engaged in some recreational marijuana use but no illicit substance use during high school. He was able to successfully complete his vocational program and subsequently find stable employment.

Final note: A strong-willed personality can sometimes be beneficial in navigating this challenging world, but children must learn to respect others, compromise, and learn restraint in order to function optimally as they mature.

HANDOUT FOR CAREGIVERS

Oppositional Defiant Disorder (ODD)

A child who is diagnosed with ODD presents with excessively argumentative and disobedient behavior, limited frustration tolerance, and anger and temper outbursts that are more intense and severe than is considered typical for their age. The first line of treatment for ODD is behavioral supports and interventions, including parent training management and individual behavioral therapy. Depending on a child's behavior at school, a child with ODD may qualify for an IEP or a 504 Accommodation Plan with school-based behavioral supports.

General Information Regarding Behavioral Issues in Children Who May or May Not Meet Criteria for a Behavioral Disorder

Attempting to figure out the possible causes of negative behaviors in children, as well as knowing how to react to these negative behaviors, can be challenging. When children are angry, they can sometimes hit, scream, swear, and slam doors. These types of behaviors can make adults uncomfortable, as they are often viewed as disrespectful, embarrassing, and even threatening. However, these behaviors are a child sending you a "signal" that something does not feel good and they do not know how to deal with the way they are feeling. An outburst can be masking underlying factors such as worry, confusion, loneliness, anxiety, jealously, or insecurity. An adult is not always able to determine what is underlying a child's behavior, but it is worth trying. While the child is cooling off in a time-out space, the adult can think about the "inside story" that may have been behind the "outside behavior" that was demonstrated by the child. Although the child's negative behaviors will continue to be considered unacceptable, it can be helpful to try to figure out if the child's "inside story" was "I'm hungry," "I'm tired," I'm feeling overwhelmed," etc., or if it is something more complex – for example, a child's history, including social challenges, over an extended period of time may result in the child reacting with an "explosion" of emotions to relatively minor incidents (Tripp, 2021).

As an adult participating in this child's life, it is important to maintain control over your own emotions. An adult cannot effectively address a child's emotional needs unless that adult is comfortable and confident in themself. Once any risk of danger is eliminated during a child's outburst, the adult needs to attempt to go beyond the anger, tears, tantrum, and physical acting out, and determine what the child is feeling and trying to communicate. We often forget that children are still developing their basic emotional vocabulary, so behavior is often the most direct way for them to communicate their discomfort.

Attempting to respond to these events in a positive manner can be challenging, but adults need to model calmness and control, and "listen" to the child's behaviors. Children need to learn more acceptable ways of communicating their needs through practicing skills that will allow them to cope with both positive and negative experiences, but these skills take time to develop. Children are impacted by what they see, hear, and experience every day from different sources, so it is important that the adult models coping skills and does not personalize a child's words or anger. As a caregiver, you are their role model, and even with your own imperfections and shortcomings, it is your responsibility to present your best self to your child during each encounter (Tripp, 2021).

Common Questions

Is my child's behavior a result of my inability to parent appropriately? Is my child just "spoiled?"
A child's behavior is related to multiple factors. Each child is "wired" a little differently and presents with their own unique character and personality. Some children are naturally more passive; some are naturally more animated; some can be more easily angered; some children may be described as more "high maintenance"; some children may frequently seek out attention, even if the attention they receive is not positive. Parenting style, however, also contributes to a child's behavioral profile. A child's specific temperament may respond differently to different parenting styles. Parents who are more easy going and less inclined to set limits may have one child who has no behavioral issues and another child who presents with challenging behaviors. Even if this child does not meet criteria for ODD, parents would likely benefit from working with a professional to learn limit setting and other techniques and strategies to help their child's behavior.

Depending on whether or not a child's difficult behavior is related to a specific mental health diagnosis, the child's temperament, and/or the parenting style used, treatment recommendations may be similar. Appropriate behaviors should be positively reinforced, and when possible, negative behaviors should be ignored. In addition, if a child's behavior is considered problematic and is negatively impacting on family life, working with a mental health professional/therapist/counselor and learning behavioral strategies that can improve the child's behavior is often beneficial.

My child has all the characteristics of ODD, but his teacher has not reported any behavioral problems in school – can he have ODD only outside of school?

It is possible that a child who only demonstrates oppositional and non-compliant behaviors at home may meet criteria for mild ODD. However, if a child demonstrates "model behavior" at school this diagnosis is less likely. Regardless of whether a specific diagnosis is definitive, the treatment would include working with a mental health professional to improve your child's behavior and social skills and help you learn appropriate behavior management strategies.

My child's tantrums are impossible to manage – sometimes she hits me or throws things at me when she's angry. Her teacher recommended that I schedule her for counseling. I did that, but all the counselor did was play with my child. She really did not seem to think that there was anything wrong with her. Now what should I do?

On one hand, when a child's counselor feels that your child does not have a mental health/behavioral diagnosis, that is good news. On the other, it does not make your job parenting your child any easier. It is important to discuss with your counselor exactly what is happening at home – even videotaping one of the episodes may be helpful. If the behaviors are only observed at home, in-home counseling/behavioral therapy can sometimes be explored. Parenting strategies that are appropriate for all children will be even more important for your child who may have a more challenging temperament.

BIBLIOGRAPHY

Achenbach T. M., & Rescorla, L.A. (2001). *Manual for the ASEBA School-Age Forms and Profiles: An Integrated System of Multi-Informant Assessment.* Burlington, Vermont: University of Vermont, Research Center for Children, Youth and Families.

Aggarwal, A., & Marwaha, R. (2022) *Oppositional Defiant Disorder.* St. Petersburg, FL: StatPearls Publishing, LLC.

American Academy of Child & Adolescent Psychiatry. www.aacap.org.

American Psychiatric Association (2013). *Diagnostic and Statistical Manual of Mental Disorders – 5th edition.* Arlington, VA: American Psychiatric Association Publishing.

American Psychiatric Association (2022). *Diagnostic and Statistical Manual of Mental Disorders – 5th edition. Text Revision.* Arlington, VA: American Psychiatric Association Publishing.

Angold, A., & Costello, E. J. (2000). The Child and Adolescent Psychiatric Assessment (CAPA). *Journal of the American Academy of Child & Adolescent Psychiatry*, 39(1): 39–48. https://doi.org/10.1097/00004583-200001000-00015.

Barkley R. A., & Benton C. M. (2013). *Your Defiant Child – 2nd edition. 8 Steps to Better Behavior.* New York, NY: The Guilford Press.

Biederman, J., Ball, S., Monuteaux, M., Kaiser, R., & Faraone, S. (2008). CBCL Clinical Scales discriminate ADHD youth with structured-interview derived diagnosis of oppositional defiant disorder (ODD). *Journal of Attention Disorders*, 12(1), 76–82. https://doi.org/10.1177/1087054707299404. Epub 2007 May 9.

Burke, J. D., Evans, S. C., & Carlson, G.A. (2022). Debate: Oppositional defiant disorder is a real disorder. *Child and Adolescent Mental Health*, 27(3): 297–299. https://doi.org/10.1111/camh.12588. Epub 2022 Jul 22.

Burke, J. D., & Loeber, R. (2017). Evidence-based interventions for oppositional defiant disorder in children and adolescents. In L. A. Theodore (Ed.), *Handbook of Evidence-Based Interventions for Children and Adolescents*: 181–191. Princeton, NJ: Springer Publishing Company.

Funderbunk, B. W., & Eyberg, S. (2011). Parent-child interaction therapy. In J. C. Norcross, G. R. VandenBos, & D. K. Freedheim (Eds.), *History of Psychotherapy: Continuity and Change – 2nd edition* (pp. 415–420). American Psychological Association. https://doi.org/10.1037/12353-021.

Goodman, R., Ford, T., Richards, H., Gatward, R., & Meltzer, H. (2000). The Development and Well-Being Assessment: Description and initial validation of an integrated assessment of child and adolescent psychopathology. *Journal of Child Psychology and Psychiatry*, 41(5): 645–655.

Grasso, M., Lazzaro, G., Demaria, F., Menghini, D., & Vicari, S. (2022). The Strengths and Difficulties Questionnaire as a valuable screening tool for identifying core symptoms and behavioural and emotional problems in children with neuropsychiatric disorders. *International Journal of Environmental Research and Public Health*, 19(13): 7731. https://doi.org/10.3390/ijerph19137731.

Greene R. W. (2021) *The Explosive Child – 6ᵗʰ edition.* New York, NY: Harper Collins Publishers.

Greene, R. W., Biederman, J., Zerwas, S., Monuteaux, M. C., Goring, J. C., Faraone, S. V. (2002). Psychiatric comorbidity, family dysfunction, and social impairment in referred youth with oppositional defiant disorder. *The American Journal of Psychiatry*, 159(7): 1214–1224. doi:10.1176/appi.ajp.159.7.1214.

Hudziak, J. J., Derks, E. M., Althoff, R. R., Copeland, W., Boomsma, D. I. (2005). The genetic and environmental contributions to oppositional defiant behavior: A multi-informant twin study. *Journal of the American Academy of Child and Adolescent Psychiatry*, 44(9): 907–914. doi: 10.1097/01.chi.0000169011.73912.27.

Jafari N., Mohammadi M. R., Khanbani M., Farid S., & Parisi C. (2011). Effect of play therapy on behavioral problems of maladjusted preschool children. *Iran Journal of Psychiatry*, 6(1): 37–42.

Kamphaus, R. W., & Reynolds, C. R. (2007). *Behavior Assessment System for Children, Second Edition (BASC-2): Behavioral and Emotional Screening System (BESS).* Bloomington, MD: Pearson.

Kazdin, A. E., Glick, A., Pope, J., Kaptchuk, T. J., Lecza, B., Carrubba, E., McWhinney, E., Hamilton. N. (2018). Parent management training for conduct problems in children: Enhancing treatment to improve therapeutic change. *Internation Journal of Clinical Health Psychology*, 18(2): 91–101. doi: 10.1016/j.ijchp.2017.12.002. Epub 2018 Feb 7.

Keenan K., & Shaw D.S. (2003). Starting at the beginning: Exploring the etiology of antisocial behavior in the first years of life. In B. B. Lahey, T. E. Moffitt, A. Caspi (Eds.), *Causes of Conduct Disorder and Juvenile Delinquency* (pp. 153–181). New York, NY: Guilford Press.

Kuny, A. V., Althoff, R. R., Copeland, W., Bartels, M., Bejsterveldt, V., Baer, J., & Hudziak, J. J. (2013). Separating the domains of oppositional behavior: Comparing latent models of the Conners' Oppositional Subscale. *Journal of the American Academy of Child and Adolescent Psychiatry*, 52(2): 172–183. https://doi.org/10.1016/j.jaac.2012.10.005.

Leadbeater, B. J., Merrin, G. J., Contreras, A., & Ames, M. E. (2023) Trajectories of oppositional defiant disorder severity from adolescence to young adulthood and substance use, mental health, and behavioral problems. *Journal of the Canadian Academy of Child and Adolescent Psychiatry*, 32(4): 224–235. Epub 2023 Nov 1.

Legha, R. K. (2025). There are no bad kids: An antiracist approach to oppositional defiant disorder. *Pediatrics*, 155(2): e2024068415. https://doi.org/10.1542/peds.2024-068415.

Leijten, P., Melendez-Torres, G., & Gardner, F. (2022). Research review: The most effective parenting program content for disruptive child behavior – A network meta-analysis. *Journal of Child Psychology and Psychiatry*, 63, 132–142. https://doi.org/10.1111/jcpp.13483. Epub 2021 Jul 9.

Lochman, J. E., Powell, N. P., Boxmeyer, C. L., Jimenez-Camargo, L. (2011). Cognitive-behavioral therapy for externalizing disorders in children and adolescents. *Child and Adolescent Psychiatry Clinics of North America*, 20(2): 305–318. https://doi.org/10.1016/j.chc.2011.01.005.

Lopez, J. D., Daniels, W., & Joshi, S. V. (2024). Oppositional defiant disorder: Clinical considerations and when to worry. *Pediatrics in Review*, 45(3): 132–142. https://doi.org/10.1542/pir.2022-005922.

Martel, M.M. (2019). *The Clinician's Guide to Oppositional Defiant Disorder: Symptoms, Assessment, and Treatment*. Cambridge, MA: Elsevier Academic Press.

Merlo, G., Chiazzese, G., Taibi, D., & Chifari, A. (2018). Development and validation of a functional behavioural assessment ontology to support behavioural health interventions. *Journal of Medical Internet Research*, 6(2), e37. https://doi.org/10.2196/medinform.7799.

Morrison, J. (2014). *DSM-5 Made Easy. The Clinician's Guide to Diagnosis*. New York, NY: The Guilford Press.

Nock, M. K., Kazdin, A. E., Hiripi, E., & Kessler, R.C. (2007). Lifetime prevalence, correlates, and persistence of oppositional defiant disorder: Results from the National Comorbidity Survey Replication. *Journal of Child Psychology and Psychiatry*, 48(7): 703–713. doi: 10.1111/j.1469-7610.2007.01733.x.

O'Laughlin, E. M., Hackenberg, J. L., & Riccardi, M. M. (2010) Clinical usefulness of the Oppositional Defiant Disorder Rating Scale (ODDRS). *Journal of Emotional and Behavioral Disorders*, 18(4): 247–255. https://doi.org/10.1177/1063426609349734.

Raine, A., Ling, S., Streicher, W., & Liu, J. (2022). The Conduct and Oppositional Defiant Disorder Scales (CODDS) for disruptive behaviour disorders. *Psychiatry Research*, 316: 11474. https://doi.org/10.1016/j.psychres.2022.114744. Epub 2022 Jul 23.

Rey, J. M., Bashir, M. R., Schwarz, M., Richards. I. N., Plapp, J. M., & Stewart, G. W. (1988). Oppositional disorder: Fact or fiction? *Journal of the American Academy of Child and Adolescent Psychiatry*, 27(2): 157–162. https://doi.org/10.1097/00004583-198803000-00004.

Riley, M., Ahmed, S., & Locke, A. (2016). Common questions about oppositional defiant disorder. *American Family Physician*, 93(7): 586–591.

Rowe, R., Costello, E. J., Angold, A., Copeland, W. E., & Maughan, B. (2011). Developmental pathways in oppositional defiant disorder and conduct disorder. *Journal of Abnormal Psychology*, 119(4):726-738. https://doi.org/10.1037/a0020798.

Rutter, M., Giller, H., & Hagell, A. (1998). *Antisocial Behavior by Young People*. New York, NY: Cambridge University Press.

Scott, S. (2022). Debate: 'A rose by any other name' would smell as sweet – myths peddled about the ills of diagnosing conduct disorders. *Child and Adolescent Mental Health*, 27(3): 302–304.

Scott, S., Briskman, J., & O'Connor, T. (2014). Early prevention of antisocial personality: Long-term follow-up of two randomized controlled trials comparing indicated and selective approaches. *American Journal of Psychiatry*, 171: 649–657. https://doi.org/10.1176/appi.ajp.2014.13050697.

Scott, S., & Gardner, F. (2015). Parent programs. In A. Thapar, D. Pine, J. Leckman, S. Scott, M. Snowling, & E. Taylor (Eds.), *Rutter's Child and Adolescent Psychiatry – 6th edition*. Oxford, England and New York, NY: Wiley Blackwell.

Shaffer, D., Fisher, P., Lucas, C. P., Dulcan, M. K., & Schwab-Stone, M. E. (2000). NIMH Diagnostic Interview Schedule for Children Version IV (NIMH DISC-IV): Description, differences from previous versions, and reliability of some common diagnoses. *Journal of the American Academy of Child and Adolescent Psychiatry*, 39: 28–38. https://doi.org/10.1097/00004583-200001000-00014.

Tripp R. (2021) *Angry kids are telling us something*. Presentation at Little People's College. New Bedford, MA.

Wise R. (2022). Five research-based interventions for oppositional defiant disorder. *https://educationalbehavior.com*.

CHAPTER 7

Learning Disorder or Just Not Trying?

Experiencing academic difficulty is not uncommon. When a child is having difficulty in school, it is important to understand if the child's poor academic performance is due to a lack of effort. For some children, academics may not come easily and may not be as enjoyable as other areas of their life; some children may experience life stressors that have a negative impact on their academic progress. However, for some children, their academic difficulties may be the result of a learning disorder.

Let us meet three children with histories of learning challenges.

CASE STUDIES

Lily always seemed bright, but in first grade her teacher reported that she was having difficulty learning to read. Her teacher recommended that she participate in the "Reading Recovery" program. By the spring of first grade, Lily made some progress, but she continued to experience challenges, and her teacher recommended that further testing be completed.

Lucas's first grade teacher reported that he was not paying attention in school. He was not following directions and seemed to be daydreaming instead of focusing on his schoolwork. A paraprofessional in the classroom began assisting Lucas and observed that he appeared anxious. As Lucas became more comfortable with the paraprofessional, she began to ask him questions about his life outside of school.

Charlotte always experienced difficulty with math and was a little socially awkward. Her parents hired a tutor for her. She worked hard and was able

DOI: 10.4324/9781003639121-7

to earn grades of As and Bs in English Language Arts (ELA) subjects and Cs in math during elementary school. She also worked with an occupational therapist to address her handwriting difficulties.

DIAGNOSIS OF A LEARNING DISABILITY/LEARNING DISORDER (LD)/SPECIFIC LEARNING DISORDER (SLD)

Please note: The terms learning disability, learning disorder, and specific learning disorder will be used interchangeably in this chapter, including the abbreviations LD and SLD.

The diagnosis of an LD involves challenges acquiring knowledge, typically academic, that are not related to a child's age, intelligence, or lack of educational opportunity. Historically an LD was defined as a significant discrepancy between an individual's intelligence quotient (IQ) and their academic ability. Standardized psychological and achievement testing were required in order for a child to be diagnosed with an LD. However, the reauthorization of the Individuals with Disabilities Act (the Individuals with Disabilities Education Improvement Act (IDEIA) of 2004) (U.S. Department of Education, 2004), specified that the identification of an LD did not need to be made utilizing the IQ-Achievement/Academic discrepancy. The law provided states with guidelines for the educational criteria for an LD and allowed school districts to utilize a student's response to research-based instruction techniques to identify students with SLDs. This method, the response to intervention (RTI) process, measures a student's response to research-based instructional methods, with the option of implementing additional research-based instructional techniques and modifications based on the student's response/resulting data (National Joint Committee on Learning Disabilities [NJCLD], 2005; Vaughn & Fuchs, 2003). The more current criteria for an LD therefore includes difficulty learning academic material, even though supports have been provided at school, or academic skills that are not appropriate for a child's age and/or grade. When making a diagnosis, one must also make sure that the child's learning challenge is not a result of an alternative diagnosis, such as an intellectual disability (ID) or visual or hearing deficit, or the results of suboptimal educational opportunities. A child's LD may be observed in only one academic area – for example, in reading (decoding, fluency, and/or comprehension), spelling, mathematics, or written language (American Psychiatric Association (APA), 2013; Morrison, 2014; Morin, 2014).

Students whose level of academic performance or rate of learning is below grade expectations are first considered "at-risk." The RTI model typically includes three tiers of intervention. Tier 1, or the primary intervention, provides instruction to students in general education classrooms. If at-risk students do not make adequate progress in Tier 1, they advance to secondary intervention, or Tier 2. Tier 2 provides students with more specialized instruction – for example, through the use of small group instruction and additional instructional time. Data regarding the student's progress are obtained in order to assess the effectiveness of the interventions. Students who do not respond adequately to Tier 1 and Tier 2 interventions, continue to Tier 3, which includes more intensive services. The student may then also qualify for a multidisciplinary evaluation to determine eligibility for an IEP (Barth et al., 2008).

AUTHORS' COMMENTARY

The following is a helpful analogy to explain an LD to children: Similar to an average or above average athlete who has difficulty in a particular sport – for example, someone who is coordinated and does well in most sports, but has always had difficulty learning to swim – an individual with a learning disability may have average or above average intelligence but experience difficulty in a specific academic area.

Evaluation

If a parent has concerns regarding their child's academic progress and suspects that the child may benefit from special education services, it is their right to request that an evaluation be completed by their school. This multidisciplinary core evaluation includes intellectual, adaptive, speech-language, and academic assessments, as well as occupational therapy, physical therapy, and social/emotional/behavioral evaluations, as indicated. Once a request for an evaluation is completed, there are federal and state law timelines that need to be followed regarding completing the evaluation. The Individuals with Disabilities Education Act (IDEA) of 2004 requires that an evaluation be completed within 60 days of the request (IDEA, 2004), but some states have laws requiring that the evaluation be completed sooner, and state laws have precedent. A parent also has the right to seek an evaluation outside their school – for example, from a university or medical center, a private learning disorders center, a psychologist, a neuropsychologist, etc.

AUTHORS' COMMENTARY

If a caregiver has concerns regarding their child's academic performance, typically the first step is to discuss the concerns with the child's teacher. If the teacher also has concerns, supports can initially be provided through the RTI program. This step-by-step approach is usually beneficial, as sometimes you may be waiting for an extended period for a full, multidisciplinary evaluation to be initiated. In addition, if the results of the full evaluation do not qualify the child for an IEP, the school is not required to complete a re-evaluation for three years. Accessing an independent evaluation can also take a long time, and can be costly, with only some insurances offering coverage.

PREVALENCE

The 2003 National Survey of Children's Health reported a prevalence estimate of learning disability of 9.7% in children aged 3–17 years old in the United States (Altarac & Saroha, 2007). The 2018–2021 data revealed a parental reported LD prevalence rate of about 8%, with a higher prevalence in boys than girls and a higher prevalence in economically disadvantaged children (Li et al., 2023).

It is worth repeating that as a result of the recognition of ethnic and socioeconomic imbalances in children who were receiving special education services, the 1997 reauthorization of IDEA included the mandate that diagnosing learning challenges should not be related to "cultural factors," "environmental or economic disadvantage," or being of "limited English proficiency." It also required that the analysis of special education data include ethnicity in order to assess the characteristics, systems, and methods that may result in disproportionate identification of children with special needs (Shifrer et al., 2011). There is a history of a disproportionate number of ethnic and racial minority students being diagnosed with learning disabilities. In an attempt to explore whether this reported disproportionality was related to "historical legacies of racism, classism, sexism, and ableism", poverty, culturally biased assessments, or other factors, Shifrer and colleagues examined patterns of identification of LD in a sample of U.S. high school students and to what extent these patterns were explained by different variables. Results suggested that a higher identification of African-American and Hispanic students with learning disabilities can be accounted for by the lower average socioeconomic status (SES) of these racial/ethnic subgroups; the diagnosis of a learning disability can be associated with a student's gender and social and demographic characteristics, as well as academic history; and being a member of a language minority can impact a student's likelihood of being diagnosed with a learning disability (Shifrer et al., 2011).

ETIOLOGY

Similar to other developmental and behavioral diagnoses, the etiology of learning disorders is considered multifactorial. A family history of learning disabilities can increase a child's risk of learning challenges. In addition, children with different types of neurologic and genetic diagnoses are considered to be at an increased risk for learning disabilities – for example, neurofibromatosis: general LD, including mathematics, reading, and difficulty with visual perceptual skills and memory; language delays/disorders: language-based learning disabilities; myelodysplasia/meningo-myelocele/spina bifida: reading comprehension, sequencing, visual-spatial and visual-motor weaknesses; Turner syndrome: non-verbal learning disability, visual-motor weaknesses; cerebral palsy: organization and sequencing, perceptual and language difficulties. Children with these types of diagnoses typically present with physical signs and other symptoms of the diagnosis, therefore it is not considered medically essential for every child who has been diagnosed with an LD to be evaluated for a neurologic or genetic diagnosis. Although there are no brain imaging studies or blood tests that can confirm or deny a diagnosis of LD, the etiology appears likely to be related to central nervous system/brain differences. A learning disorder can therefore be considered a neuro-developmental diagnosis, and this places a child with LD at an increased risk for other developmental-behavioral challenges.

DIFFERENT "TYPES" OF LD

Children who are diagnosed with a **language-based learning disorder** present with difficulty in language-based academic subjects, typically reading, written expression, and spelling. Early oral language has been reported to be predictive of later reading comprehension ability (Butler et al., 1985; Milburn et al., 2017; Storch & Whitehurst, 2002), and phonological awareness and knowledge of letters have been reported to be associated with later decoding ability (Lonigan et al., 2008). Young children struggling with acquisition of language-based skills may therefore be at increased risk for future language-based learning challenges. However, it is important to note that the future of children with speech-language delays and disorders is variable – some disorders resolve; some persist or change characteristic (for example, an expressive language disorder or speech/articulation disorder can later present as a disorder of speech fluency); while some of these children later present with a language-based learning disability.

Because identification of children at risk for language-based LD typically focused on school-aged children, Milburn and colleagues assessed whether the methods of identifying LD in school-aged children could be used to predict which preschoolers may be at risk for future language-based learning challenges. Children were classified as "at risk" based on three early-literacy skills – language, phonological awareness, and print knowledge. A comparison of four methods of determining LD was completed in 1,011 preschool children – IQ-achievement discrepancy; poor achievement/academic performance; poor academic growth; combination of two methods. Results revealed poor rates of agreement among the methods, suggesting that identifying young children who may be at risk for future learning disorders can be challenging (Milburn et al., 2017).

Children with a **non-verbal learning disability** (this was sometimes previously referred to as a "right hemispheric learning disability") present with difficulty in non-language based cognitive and academic areas – these may include visual-spatial challenges and problems with mathematics, as well as additional social and motor difficulties.

LEARNING DISORDERS CAN ALSO BE CATEGORIZED BASED ON SPECIFIC ACADEMIC CHALLENGES

Specific LD With Impairment in Reading – Also Historically Referred to as Dyslexia

This diagnosis is based on a child's inability to learn to read at the level expected for the child's age and intelligence. It is important to note that learning to read, i.e., developing an understanding of the written word, is based on the ability to decode words together with language comprehension. Difficulty with either of these skills can result in reading difficulty. A specific reading disorder can include challenges in decoding, comprehension, oral reading, and/or accuracy of reading. The diagnosis of dyslexia often brings to mind letter reversals, for example, misreading a "b" for a "d"; although this can be a characteristic in children who have difficulty with decoding/using phonics to sound out words, the term dyslexia currently refers to any reading disorder, whether or not the child is reported to often demonstrate reversals of letters/numbers.

Specific LD With Impairment in Mathematics – Dyscalculia

For some children, mathematics is a more difficult subject for them than reading and writing. Sometimes the difficulty is severe enough to meet criteria for the diagnosis of dyscalculia. As stated above, sometimes dyscalculia can be one of the presenting signs of a nonverbal learning disability.

Specific LD with Impairment in Written Expression

Some children present with specific difficulties with grammar, punctuation, spelling, and/or putting their thoughts into writing.

CASE STUDIES

Despite the support in reading and writing that **Lily** received through the RTI program, she continued to struggle. An evaluation was completed by her school. Results of cognitive testing revealed an IQ in the average range. Lily's non-language-based skills on IQ testing were above average and her language-based skills were below average. Results of educational testing revealed a significant weakness in Lily's reading and written language scores. Lily was diagnosed with SLDs in reading and written Expression. The diagnosis of language-based learning disability was also included in the psychologist's report.

Lucas had psychoeducational testing completed and his scores were average, although his score in written language was at the lower end of the average range. Lucas informed the paraprofessional that his family had changed their home frequently and for a period of time were living in a shelter.

Charlotte's parents and her teacher felt that a multidisciplinary evaluation should be completed. The evaluation included psycho-educational testing and an occupational therapy evaluation. Charlotte was diagnosed with a non-verbal learning disorder and fine and visual-motor skill weaknesses and qualified for an IEP.

EMOTIONAL ISSUES

Psycho-social and emotional issues can have a negative impact on academic performance. Conversely, difficulty in school can be associated with a lowering of a child's self-esteem and sometimes frustration, which can lead to decreased motivation and limited attention span, and sometimes behavioral problems (Arnold & Doctoroff, 2003; Milburn et al., 2017). Identifying and intervening earlier for children who are at risk for academic difficulties can be beneficial in attempting to avoid these associated challenges (Milburn et al., 2017).

THE COVID-19 PANDEMIC

The intensity and complexity of the impact of the COVID-19 pandemic on educational systems and on students of all ages cannot be overemphasized. Students' educational achievement was negatively impacted by the pandemic, and not surprisingly, socioeconomically disadvantaged students were disproportionately impacted. Gee and colleagues reviewed research examining "disparate educational impacts of the pandemic across racial, ethnic, and socioeconomic status groups that deepened existing educational inequities in the United States." The study reported "disparate access to full-time in-person learning across racial/ethnic groups among U.S. K–12 students over the 2020–21 school year, by geography and school level. The populations with the most access to full-time in-person learning were non-Hispanic White students, students living in the South, and those in grades K–5" (Gee et al., 2023).

AUTHORS' COMMENTARY

We observed the multifaceted effects the pandemic had on the families in our practices. The impact of social isolation, virtual learning, family stress, and financial and health burdens, cannot be overstated. The use of technology and "screen time" increased during the pandemic with children spending numerous hours each day interfacing with electronic devices, including virtual learning. Children had less opportunity for social interaction and peer-to-peer academic work. The long-term effects of the COVID-19 pandemic on children's development will require ongoing research and follow-up. Consideration of "pandemic factors" should be part of assessing children's developmental and learning profiles.

CHILDREN WHO HAVE ACADEMIC DIFFICULTIES BUT DO NOT MEET CRITERIA FOR AN SLD

If results of testing reveal some weaknesses but are not suggestive of a specific learning disability, and a child has responded to educational supports at school, i.e., the child does not meet criteria for an LD, the child may still continue to experience academic challenges. It is still therefore important to provide the child with supports both at school and outside of school in order to prevent academics becoming a negative experience, lowering the child's self-esteem, and setting the child up for future problems. Academic supports that are available to all children can be explored, such as after school assistance programs or tutoring outside of school. The wide range of cognitive abilities, social and family backgrounds, and academic skills of children who do not qualify for an IEP are important to acknowledge. These children also require support throughout their educational experience.

AUTHOR'S COMMENTARY

Academic Underachievement

There are a multitude of reasons why a child may not be performing in line with their academic potential. It is important to rule out an ID and an LD as the etiology of a child's suboptimal academic performance. Other diagnoses that are important to consider include attention-deficit/hyperactivity disorder (ADHD) and other mental health diagnoses – for example, anxiety and depression. Family stress can also contribute to a child's suboptimal academic performance; if a child is sleeping poorly, is worried about the well-being of family members, has poor nutrition and is frequently feeling hungry, or has developed a feeling of poor self-esteem (a feeling that they are unintelligent and will "never" be as smart as his/her peers), then their academic performance is likely to be compromised. It is not infrequent for a parent to question whether the etiology of a child's suboptimal academic performance is "boredom", i.e., the academic work is too "easy" for them, so does not keep their interest. Although it is important to consider whether a child may require more challenging work, in the authors' experiences, children who have strong cognitive and academic skills may independently seek out more challenging work after quickly completing the required work in school. Finally, if a child does not show an interest in academics – for example, if they are more of a "hands-on" learner – ways to make academics more enjoyable for them should be explored.

EDUCATIONAL TECHNIQUES TO HELP FACILITATE LEARNING (TRIPP, 2022)

- Children are acquiring new knowledge all the time. Instructors need to review foundational information every day, multiple times a day. Reviewing information on a daily basis helps the information to become part of a child's memory. This strategy is applicable to both academic information and behavioral rules. Consequences of not following rules should also be reviewed frequently. ("Cramming" information is not a good teaching strategy.) It is often easiest to recall the first and last thing you hear. Therefore, discussing specific ideas and instructions first thing in the morning, reviewing them throughout the day, and recapping the information at the end of the day can help facilitate retention.
- Having students repeat information, initially aloud and later internally, can be beneficial. Student may need to be taught to identify important information they should rehearse, as repeating rote information word-for-word is less helpful.
- Alternating between old and new content can also be beneficial. If something new is introduced to the children, it can be helpful to connect it to something that they have already learned.
- When you combine words with visuals that are meaningful, children have two ways to understand the information and it becomes more concrete to them. Children need enough time to absorb the visuals and the verbal explanation. Use of multiple modalities – auditory, visual, kinesthetic – can assist in facilitating learning.
- The use of social stories can help children develop connections between visual and verbal instruction. Remember, what is meaningful is memorable.
- Try to limit distractions. Scheduling breaks is important, but attempt to avoid a break in the middle of a lesson if possible. Taking breaks at a crucial teaching time can derail children's focus. It is challenging to get a group back on track once they have been interrupted.
- It is typically easier to recall information when it is grouped into more manageable "chunks" – for example, "58-23-86" is easier to recall than "5-8-2-3-8-6.
- Acronyms are used from childhood through adulthood to help remember specific information – for example, call the "COPS" to help remember to check Capitalization, Overall appearance, Punctuation, and Spelling when proofreading.

AUTHORS' COMMENTARY

It is important to reiterate that the skill of reading requires the ability to use phonics to sound out words/decode, in combination with language comprehension. Research has shown that using pictures to "guess" a word, which was one technique included in the previous "balanced literacy/whole language" approach to reading, is not currently considered "best practice." (Seidenberg, 2017)

Specialized Instruction for Children with LDs

In addition to the techniques discussed above, there are specialized instructional programs that can be used to teach children who have been diagnosed with a learning disorder. Teaching programs, strategies, and supports for children who are experiencing learning challenges have provoked controversies and different "schools of thought" throughout history. Reviewing specific strategies and programs is beyond the scope of this book, but we chose to briefly mention two programs that we have seen used in school systems during our careers. The **Orton-Gillingham approach** is a multisensory, structured, sequential, technique to teach reading, writing, and spelling. The program was based on the contributions of Samuel T. Orton, a neuropsychologist and pathologist, and Anna Gillingham, an educator and psychologist (National Center for Educational Statistics, 2010). The **Wilson Reading System** is a systemic, multisensory and interactive approach that teaches word structure for decoding and encoding (Orton-Gillingham principles are incorporated into the program) (Wilson & Wilson, 1988).

Auditory Perceptual Deficits/Central Auditory Processing (CAP) Disorder

Children with auditory processing challenges can appear to have a hearing deficit, but testing will reveal normal hearing bilaterally. These children can experience difficulty understanding information presented to them verbally. They can also experience more difficulty when background noise is present. Specific testing can be completed by an audiologist to assess for a CAP disorder. The diagnosis will typically qualify a student for accommodations in school. Some strategies that can be helpful for children with a CAP disorder include:

- providing preferential seating close to the teacher;
- attempting to reduce background noise;

- if possible, scheduling activities that require more intensive listening skills earlier during the school day;
- getting a child's attention, prior to giving instructions;
- repeating and rephrasing instructions and supplementing instructions with visual materials;
- assessing a child's comprehension of instructions by confirming their understanding.

CASE STUDIES

An IEP was created and **Lily** received academic assistance with a special education teacher, including a reading specialist. She responded well to the Orton-Gillingham specialized reading program and made progress in her skills. She was provided with some accommodations in science and social studies in higher grades – Lily's ability to understand social studies and science was above her grade level, so she was provided with audio recordings of the written material.

Lucas began to meet with the school counselor who contacted social services. Lucas's family was provided with assistance and supports, and they were able to find more permanent housing. Lucas's functioning in school gradually improved, and his academics remained at grade level.

Charlotte's IEP included academic assistance in math and occupational therapy. She also participated in a social skills group. It was also notable that Charlotte's medical history was significant for short stature. She had an endocrinology consultation and results of chromosome testing was consistent with the diagnosis of Turner syndrome. Charlotte continued to be followed by an endocrinologist.

MEDICATION?

Medication is not used to treat a learning disability, unless another disorder co-exists – for example, ADHD, anxiety, depression.

CASE STUDIES

Lily did well in high school and went to college. Some accommodations continued to be implemented – for example, she continued to supplement some of her books in college with audio books. Lily incorporated her life experiences into her career as a special education teacher.

Charlotte continued to be followed by an endocrinologist. She attended college and majored in journalism. As an adult she worked for a newspaper and wrote a personal blog about her diagnosis and her associated learning disability.

Final note: It is important to understand a child's strengths and weaknesses so the child can utilize and facilitate their strengths and work on improving their areas of weakness.

HANDOUT FOR CAREGIVERS

The diagnosis of an learning disability/learning disorder (LD) includes difficulty learning academic material despite supports that have been provided at school, or academic skills below what is considered age and grade appropriate and that have a negative impact on a child's academic progress and school experience. In addition, the learning/academic difficulties are not caused by an alternative diagnosis such as an intellectual disability (ID) or visual or hearing deficit, and are not a result of limited access to appropriate educational opportunities. A child's LD may be observed in only one academic area, – for example, in reading (decoding, fluency, and/or comprehension), spelling, mathematics, or written language (American Psychiatric Association, 2013; Morrison, 2014; Morin, 2014).

Common Questions

My child is struggling at school. What is the best and possibly quickest way to have my child evaluated for a learning disorder?
If you have a concern regarding your child's academic progress, the best place to start exploring a path forward is to discuss your concerns with your child's teacher. The teacher can often provide some insight regarding your child's skills compared to what is expected at the current grade level. If you or your child's teacher feels that your child may benefit from special education services, you can request that an evaluation be completed by the school. Once a request for an evaluation is completed, there are federal and state law timelines that need to be followed regarding completing the evaluation. You also have the right to seek an evaluation outside the school – for example, from a medical center, a private learning disorders center, a psychologist, a neuropsychologist, etc. However, you should first explore the cost and whether the evaluation will be covered by your child's health insurance. Having the evaluation completed in a timely manner can sometimes be frustrating, so placing your child's name on multiple cancellation lists may result in them being seen sooner. Finally, other parents and local advocacy groups may be helpful when exploring resources in your community.

Is there a cure for my child's learning disability?
Educational programs and supports are the treatment for a learning disability. Children who receive special education typically show improvement in their academic achievement. Whether a child is eventually able to perform at grade level may depend on the severity of their learning disability.

BIBLIOGRAPHY

Alabbad, M., Khan, M. A., Siddique, N., Hassan, J. A., Bashir, S., & Abu-alait, T. (2023). Early predictors in language-based learning disabilities: A bibliometric analysis. *Frontiers in Psychiatry*, 14: 1229580. https://doi.org/10.3389/fpsyt.2023.1229580.

Altarac, M., & Saroha, E. (2007). Lifetime prevalence of learning disability among US children. *Pediatrics*, 119: S77–S83. https://doi.org/10.1542/peds.2006-2089L.

Al-Yagon, M., Cavendish, W., Cornoldi, C., Fawcett, A. J., Grünke, M., Hung, L. Y., Jimenez, J. E., Karande, S., van Kraayenoord, C. E., Lucangeli, D., Margalit, M., Montague, M., Sholapurwala, R., Sideridis, G., Tressoldi, P. E., & Vio, C. (2013). The proposed changes for DSM-5 for SLD and ADHD: International perspectives – Australia, Germany, Greece, India, Israel, Italy, Spain, Taiwan, United Kingdom, and United States. *Journal of Learning Disabilities*, 46: 58–72. https://doi.org/10.1177/0022219412464353.

American Psychiatric Association (APA) (2013). *Diagnostic and Statistical Manual of Mental Disorders – 5th edition*. Arlington, VA: American Psychiatric Association Publishing.

Arnold, D. H., & Doctoroff, G. L. (2003). The early education of socioeconomically disadvantaged children. *Annual Review of Psychology*, 54: 517–545. https://doi.org/10.1146/annurev.psych.54.111301.145442. Epub 2002 Jun 10.

Barth, A. E., Stuebing, K. K., Anthony, J. L., Denton, C. A., Mathes, P. G., Fletcher, J. M., & Francis, D. J. (2008). Agreement among response to intervention criteria for identifying responder status. *Learning and Individual Differences*, 18(3): 296–307. https://doi.org/10.1016/j.lindif.2008.04.004.

Butler, S. R., Marsh, H. W., Sheppard, M. J., & Sheppard, J. L. (1985). Seven-year longitudinal study of the early prediction of reading achievement. *Journal of Educational Psychology*, 77: 349–361. https://doi.org/10.1037/0022-0663.77.3.349.

Dyscalculia.org. www.dyscalculia.org.

Gee, K. A., Asmundson, V., & Vang, T. (2023). Educational impacts of the COVID-19 pandemic in the United States: Inequities by race, ethnicity, and socioeconomic status. *Current Opinion in Psychology*, 52: 101643. https://doi.org/10.1016/j.copsyc.2023.101643. Epub 2023 Jul 11.

Individuals with Disabilities Education Act (IDEA) (2004). 20 U.S.C. Section 1400.

LD Online. www.ldonline.org.

Learning Disabilities Association of America. www.ldaamerica.org.

Li, Q., Li, Y., Zheng, J., Yan, X., Huang, J., Xu, Y., Zeng, X., Shen, T., Xing, X., Chen, Q., & Yang, W. (2023). Prevalence and trends of developmental disabilities among US children and adolescents aged 3 to 17 years, 2018–2021. *Scientific Reports*,13(1): 17254. https://doi.org/10.1038/s41598-023-44472-1.

Lonigan, C. J., Schatschneider, C., & Westberg, L. (2008). *Developing early literacy: Report of the national early literacy panel* (pp. 55–106). Washington, D.C.: National Institute for Literacy.

Milburn, T. F., Lonigan, C. J., Allan, D. M., & Phillips, B. M. (2017). Agreement among traditional and RTI-based definitions of reading-related learning disability with preschool children. *Learning and Individual Differences*, April(55): 120–129. https://doi.org/10.1016/j.lindif.2017.03.011.

Morin, A. (2014). *The Everything Parent's Guide to Special Education*. New York, NY: Simon and Schuster.

Morrison, J. (2014). *DSM-5 Made Easy. The Clinician's Guide to Diagnosis*. New York: NY: The Guilford Press.

National Center for Education Statistics (2010). *Orton-Gillingham-based strategies*. www.nces.ed.gov.

National Center for Learning Disabilities. www.ncld.org.

National Joint Committee on Learning Disabilities (NJCLD) (2005). *Responsiveness to intervention and learning disabilities: A report prepared by the National Joint Committee on Learning Disabilities representing eleven national and international organizations*. Washington, D.C.

Reading Rockets. www.readingrockets.org.

Seidenberg, M. (2017). *Language at the Speed of Sight: How We Read, Why So Many Can't, and What Can Be Done About It*. New York, NY: Basic Books.

Shifrer, D., Muller, C., & Callahan, R. (2011) Disproportionality and learning disabilities: Parsing apart race, socioeconomic status, and language. *Journal of Leaning Disabilities*, 44(3): 246–257. https://doi.org/10.1177/0022219410374236.

Storch, S. A., & Whitehurst, G. J. (2002). Oral language and code-related precursors to reading: Evidence from a longitudinal structural model. *Developmental Psychology*, 38: 934–947.

Tripp R. (2022). *The science of learning*. Presentation at Little People's College. New Bedford, MA.

U.S. Department of Education (1975). *Individuals with Disabilities Act (IDEA)* https://sites.ed.gov.

U.S. Government (2004). Individuals With Disabilities Education Improvement Act of 2004 (Public Law No. 108-446). www.govinfo.gov/app/details/PLAW-108publ446.

Vaughn S., & Fuchs L. S. (2003). Redefining learning disabilities as inadequate response to instruction: The promise and potential problems. *Learning Disabilities Research & Practice*, 18(3): 137–146. https://doi.org/10.1111/1540-5826.00070.

Wilson B., & Wilson E. (1988). *Wilson Reading System (WRS)*. Wilson Langugae Training. https://www.wilsonlanguage.com/programs/wilson-reading-system/.

CHAPTER 8

Anxiety Disorder or Just Really Cautious?

Feelings of worry, anxiety, and fearfulness are experienced by everyone. In fact, feeling a little bit anxious can sometimes be beneficial – it may prevent a child from doing something dangerous, or it may be helpful for an adolescent in preparing for an exam or a presentation. In addition, worrying about negative occurrences such as crime and school shootings are unfortunately acceptable current concerns. But when is worrying considered a problem? An anxiety disorder is characterized by an intense amount of fear and anxiety that has a negative impact on a person's functioning. In addition to being considered its own group of mental health disorders, it is also important to note that anxiety may be associated with other mental health and developmental disorders.

Let us meet Aurora, Mateo, and Ava.

CASE STUDIES

Aurora is four years old, and she has always been somewhat shy. Aurora's mother reported that there were previously no significant concerns about Aurora's development, with the exception of some mild delays in her speech. By the time Aurora was evaluated by a speech therapist when she was two-and-a-half years old, it was felt that her communication skills were age-appropriate. During Aurora's first year of preschool it was reported that Aurora was not talking when she was at school. It was initially felt that Aurora's silence at school was related to her shyness in combination with this being her first experience in a school environment. However, after nine months Aurora is still not speaking to any of the teachers and has not been heard to verbally communicate with the other students. Aurora responds to

DOI: 10.4324/9781003639121-8

requests made by the other students, and plays quietly with them, but for the most part she is silent throughout the school day. At home, Aurora continues to speak with family members. Aurora's teachers are concerned, and her mother has requested advice.

Mateo is three years old. He has always appeared somewhat cautious. During his first playground visit, he was fearful of using the slide; however, with encouragement, he was finally willing to go up and down the slide on his mother's lap. During Mateo's third visit to the playground, with encouragement and "cheering," he was willing to use the slide independently. When meeting new people, Mateo often hides behind his mother. Finally, Mateo is fearful of insects. He will play outside, but if he sees an insect, he will run away and look for "protection" from a parent. Mateo's parents are concerned that Mateo may have an anxiety disorder.

Ava is seven years old. She has consistently had one or two close friends at school. There were previously no concerns regarding her social skills or behavior. However, in the middle of second grade, Ava began to resist attending school. She cries and even sometimes demonstrates a tantrum saying she no longer wants to go to school. After arriving at school, she holds her head down on her desk and does not participate. Ava frequently complains of stomach aches; she asks to go to the nurse and then asks them to call her mother to pick her up and take her home.

ANXIETY DISORDERS

There are several types of anxiety disorders, and together they are considered one of the most frequently occurring mental health diagnoses. For example, an anxiety disorder can be considered "general"; related to social situations; or related to a specific fear/"phobia" (American Psychiatric Association [APA], 2013; Morrison, 2014). It is not unusual for children to exhibit anxiety. Afterall, they are having new and unfamiliar experiences on a regular basis, and they are working on developing the skills to manage everyday experiences that may be frightening or unsettling. However, anxiety is considered a disorder when a child's persistent worrying/fears over an extended period of time cause an abnormally high amount of distress and impede the child from being able to appropriately engage in age-appropriate activities. A child's anxiety may be associated with other signs/symptoms – for example, abdominal discomfort, vomiting, extreme outbursts, sleep difficulties, and avoidance of participation in age-appropriate activities (APA, 2013; Morrison, 2014).

PREVALENCE AND DEMOGRAPHICS

Anxiety disorders are relatively common, with prevalence estimates of between 5 and 12% of children and adolescents (Rapee et al., 2023). Reports regarding demographics have been variable, with no definitive association between socioeconomic status or parental education and risk for anxiety disorders (Rapee et al., 2023). The most consistent demographic association is gender, with females at higher risk for anxiety disorders than males, with an increase in gender discrepancy beginning during puberty (Khanal et al., 2022; Rapee et al., 2023; Vicente et al., 2012).

RISK FACTORS

A **family history** of anxiety and/or mood disorders increases a child's risk for anxiety disorders (Lawrence et al., 2019; Lee et al., 2021; Penninx et al., 2021; Rapee, et al., 2023). It has also been reported that certain anxiety disorders (for example, generalized anxiety disorder) carry a stronger genetic influence than some others types of anxiety disorders (Waszczuk et al., 2014). In addition, mood disorders, including depression, can share a genetic risk with anxiety disorders (Penninx, et al., 2021).

There has been research in molecular genetics and neurophysiology (specifically functioning brain scans) exploring both the contributions of specific genes to the heritability of anxiety disorders, as well as possible central nervous system differences via neuroimaging. Functional brain scans examine the activity levels in different areas of the brain, "mapping" brain activity. Any positive results from studies of functional brain scans and genetic studies have so far suggested relationships with general psychopathology rather than a direct relationship between atypical findings and specific mental health disorders, including anxiety (Rapee, et al., 2023).

There has been research regarding the relationship between a child's temperament and risk of anxiety. A child's temperament indicates certain personal behavioral traits – for example, a child may be described as "rigid," "irritable," "easygoing," or "high strung." Studies have examined personal traits such as a tendency toward withdrawal, shyness, fearfulness, and what has been termed "behavioral inhibition" as possible risk factors for anxiety (Liu & Bell, 2020; Rapee et al., 2009). Behavioral inhibition refers to the avoidance of novel, unfamiliar events (Kagan et al., 1984). It is notable that a high physical and emotional reactivity to novel stimuli has been reported as being observed as early as three months of age (Fox et al., 2015; Kagan et al., 1998), and has been reported to increase a child's risk of later behavioral inhibition. However, the possibility that behavioral inhibition is a characteristic of anxiety rather than a distinct behavioral trait has also been proposed (Rapee & Coplan, 2010). Overall, there are still many unanswered questions regarding the relationship between temperament and anxiety.

Environmental factors have also been proposed as risk factors for anxiety, including parenting style, peer relationships, negative life experiences, and school experiences. Overprotective parenting, parent modeling of anxious behaviors, and over-controlling parenting have all been hypothesized as possibly contributing to childhood anxiety (Rapee et al., 2023). However, results of research on parenting style as a risk factor have been variable, and genetic risk can act as a confounding variable, i.e., parental anxiety disorder can increase a child's risk of anxiety. Negative school experiences and social challenges, including bullying and academic difficulty with associated poor self-esteem, as well as negative life experiences, have all been considered as factors that may contribute to childhood anxiety (Rapee et al., 2023).

MEDICAL DIAGNOSES

Medical diagnoses that cause or contribute to a child's anxiety are also important to consider.

- Thyroid dysfunction, particularly hyperthyroidism, can be associated with anxiety; however, it is typically associated with other signs and symptoms in addition to anxiety;
- As discussed above, some genetic disorders, and central nervous system abnormalities, can increase a child's risk for some mental health diagnoses, including anxiety;
- Chronic medical conditions can be associated with an increased risk of anxiety – for example, a child or adolescent with inflammatory bowel disease, may start to worry excessively that their condition may result in a soiling accident at school;
- Certain medications can increase a child's risk of presenting with anxiety-type symptoms – for example, steroids and some asthma and allergy medications.

DIAGNOSING ANXIETY DISORDER

Similar to other mental health diagnoses, the diagnosis of an anxiety disorder is based on a child's history and clinical presentation, with confirmation of the diagnosis made by an experienced professional. There are self-report, clinician-report, parent-report, and teacher-report questionnaires and checklists available that can assist a clinician in assessing for anxiety – for example, the Multidimensional Anxiety Scale for Children (MASC) (self-report) (March et al.,1997); Screen for Child Anxiety Related Disorders (SCARED) (self-report and parent report) (Birmaher, et al., 1997); Achenbach Child Behavior Checklist (CBCL) – Parent and Teacher (Achenbach & Rescorla, 2001); and Pediatric Anxiety Rating Scale (PARS) (Riddle et al., 2002). Results of these types of questionnaires can contribute valuable diagnostic information that can assist in determining whether further evaluation is needed.

When is Anxiety Considered "Normal?"

It is important to note that many childhood fears are age-appropriate. For example, infants experience "stranger anxiety," and "separation anxiety" is demonstrated by typically developing toddlers as they prefer to stay near familiar adults (see Chapter 1). Certain fears are typical at certain ages. A preschooler may be fearful of "monsters," the dark, or "scary dreams"; an elementary school child may be afraid of a "kidnapper" or natural disasters that they have heard about on TV; preadolescents may fear not being as good as their peers and are concerned about being made fun of. Some children are "naturally" more anxious than others – for example, a child who may be considered bright and thoughtful may "think" about potentially dangerous things longer and harder than other children. These types of fears are considered within the range of typical childhood development. Helping a child work through these types of age-appropriate fears is beneficial, as it will help them learn skills to deal with other anxiety provoking situations as they mature.

Differential Diagnosis and Co-Morbid Diagnoses

Anxiety can be a characteristic of, and/or overlap with, symptoms of other diagnoses. In addition, anxiety disorder can occur co-morbidly with other mental health diagnoses. Having a specific anxiety disorder increases an individual's risk for other types of anxiety disorders, as well as other mental health diagnoses, sometimes concurrently, and sometimes in the future. It is notable that children who have been diagnosed with more than one type of anxiety disorder and/or co-morbid mental health diagnoses have been reported to typically experience more functional impairment than those diagnosed with a single anxiety disorder (Cummings et al., 2014; Rapee et al., 2013).

Depression

This diagnosis is discussed in Chapter 9. Children whose primary diagnosis is depression can also experience poor concentration, sleep difficulties, somatic complaints, tension and anxiety (i.e., their symptoms may overlap with symptoms of anxiety). In addition, it is not uncommon for a diagnosis of depression to occur co-morbidly with an anxiety disorder, especially in adolescents (Costello et al., 2003; Cummings et al., 2014; Khanal et al., 2022). It has been reported that approximately 10 to 15% of clinically anxious children and adolescents also meet diagnostic criteria for a mood disorder (Cummings et al., 2014).

Autism Spectrum Disorder (ASD)

This diagnosis is discussed in Chapter 4. Children with ASD are at increased risk for anxiety – for example, a change in routine can provoke anxiety. A child with ASD who is demonstrating ongoing, significant anxiety may also meet criteria for an anxiety disorder. Although it can sometimes be challenging to differentiate a co-morbid diagnosis of an anxiety disorder from anxiety being a characteristic of ASD, some studies have reported a relatively high rate of comorbidity (Lai et al., 2019; Rapee, et al., 2023).

Attention-Deficit/Hyperactivity Disorder (ADHD) and Oppositional Defiant Disorder (ODD)

The diagnosis of ADHD is discussed in Chapter 5, and the diagnosis of ODD is discussed in Chapter 6. Children with ADHD often present as restless and inattentive, which can also be characteristics of anxiety. Similar to other mental health diagnoses, anxiety disorders can occur co-morbidly with externalizing disorders, including ADHD and ODD (Rapee et al., 2023).

AUTHORS' COMMENTARY

Anxiety and depression can sometimes be categorized as "internalizing" disorders, presenting with worry, sadness, decreased interest in participating in activities, poor sleep, abnormalities in eating patterns, etc. However, children who are worried, fearful, or sad, can also "externalize" those feelings by acting out and presenting as irritable and overly active. It is therefore important to consider whether a child who is presenting with features of ADHD or ODD may be presenting with an anxiety disorder as their primary diagnosis.

Posttraumatic Stress Disorder (PTSD)

This diagnosis is discussed in Chapter 11. Anxiety is a key characteristic of PTSD, a disorder that can develop after experiencing a traumatic event. When a child presents with anxiety, it is always important to explore a child's family and social history in detail, with ongoing exploration over time, as a history of trauma may take time to uncover.

Obsessive-Compulsive Disorder (OCD)

This diagnosis is discussed in Chapter 10. Experiencing obsessive and/or compulsive thoughts and/or behaviors can be associated with anxiety.

AUTHORS' COMMENTARY

It is important to note that in addition to the risk of co-morbid psychopathology, a child with an anxiety disorder (particularly if untreated) can be at risk for academic and social problems.

CASE STUDIES

Aurora's parents discussed Aurora's preschool issues with her pediatrician, who felt that Aurora was presenting with the diagnosis of selective mutism. An audiology assessment was completed, and Aurora was tested to have normal hearing. The pediatrician referred Aurora to a therapist for further evaluation. The therapist confirmed the diagnosis of selective mutism and began using positive reinforcement and play to encourage Aurora to verbalize, initially with the therapist and eventually at school.

 Mateo had an evaluation with a counselor. He demonstrated some age-appropriate fears, but he was also considered more anxious than many children his age. However, it was not felt that he met criteria for an anxiety disorder, as his fears were age-appropriate and resolved relatively quickly with support. The counselor worked with Mateo and his parents to explore ways to address Mateo's fears. Mateo continued to be a fairly cautious child and demonstrated what were considered age-appropriate fears throughout childhood. His teachers and the school counselor were notified of his history and monitored him for anxiety-related issues. Mateo enjoyed nature –

walking on nature trails (even with the insects), and art-related activities proved to be very therapeutic for him. It was never felt that he met criteria for an anxiety disorder.

When **Ava** was at the school nurse's office, the nurse began asking Ava about her family. Ava reported that she loved being at home. She also reported that her pet had died at the end of first grade, and she still cried a lot as she thought about him "all the time." A meeting was scheduled that included Ava's parents, the school nurse, the school psychologist, and the school counselor. Ava's mother confided that she was previously treated with medication for an anxiety disorder. There were concerns that Ava may be presenting with an anxiety disorder, and she was referred for a consultation with a therapist outside of school.

TREATMENT

Behavioral therapy is recommended for children with anxiety, and collaboration is needed among the child's family members, therapists, and school staff. Behavioral therapy often involves cognitive behavioral therapy (CBT) and, depending on the age and specific diagnosis of the child, play therapy and/or other therapies may be recommended. Medications can also be used to treat anxiety, although less frequently in children than in adolescents and adults.

CBT

Cognitive behavioral therapy is the most extensively researched and implemented intervention used to treat pediatric anxiety disorders (Dickson et al., 2022; Rapee et al., 2023). CBT was discussed in previous chapters but is worth reviewing. CBT includes:

- identifying precipitants of stress;
- learning to better understand the disorder ("psychoeducation");
- learning to replace stress-producing thoughts and actions with non-stress producing thoughts and actions ("cognitive restructuring");
- gradual and structured desensitization using imagery and exposure to precipitants;
- modification of behavior using positive rewards and elimination of negative stimuli ("operant conditioning");
- implementation of relaxation techniques.

Benefits of CBT for treatment of childhood anxiety disorders have been consistently reported for children of various ages and ethnicities, and across various cultures (Rapee et al., 2022a). The 2020 Cochrane review provided some evidence of efficacy of CBT for treatment of childhood anxiety disorders. Some of the reported limitations of the 88 randomized controlled trials included limited research in children less than eight years old and children with additional special needs (James et al., 2020). There has been some evidence that CBT may be less effective for treatment of a social anxiety disorder vs. other anxiety disorders (Evans et al., 2021). However, there have been some relatively recent reports regarding methods of improving outcomes of CBT for treatment of social anxiety, including implementation of a "modified disorder-specific" form of CBT (Rapee et al., 2022a), that targets the specific psychological processes believed to maintain social anxiety disorder (Rapee et al., 2022a; Rapee et al., 2022b).

AUTHORS' COMMENTARY

Relaxation exercises can be a part of CBT – for example, deep, slow breathing exercises. It is worth noting that physical exercise – for example, yoga, swimming, and dance – can provide relaxation and can assist in reducing anxiety, whether or not a child meets criteria for an anxiety disorder.

Pharmacotherapy

Although behavioral therapy is typically considered the first line of treatment for children with anxiety, sometimes a trial of treatment with medication may be indicated. Selective serotonin reuptake inhibitors (SSRIs) are sometimes used to treat childhood anxiety. Selective serotonin reuptake inhibitors work by limiting the reabsorption of the neurotransmitter serotonin, thereby increasing the extracellular levels of serotonin. However, the use of SSRIs in young children needs to be approached with caution. For example, although sertraline has been shown to be effective in treating pediatric anxiety (Wang et al., 2017), it has only been approved by the Food and Drug Administration (FDA) for treatment of OCD in children aged six years and older (see Chapter 10). Similarly, other SSRI medications have been approved for children aged seven or eight years and older who have been diagnosed with depression (Chapter 9) or OCD (Chapter 10) (Hussain et al., 2016). Serotonin-norepinephrine reuptake inhibitors (SNRIs) have also been used to treat anxiety, one of which received relatively recent FDA approval for treatment of generalized anxiety disorder in children. Other medications that have sometimes been prescribed by psychiatrists to treat pediatric anxiety disorders have included antidepressant medications, benzodiazepine medications, and some anticonvulsant/anti-epileptic medications (Penninx et al., 2021; Strawn et al., 2021), but these have not been used as frequently of SSRIs and SNRIs.

CBT and SSRI

Although research has revealed variable results when comparing CBT to treatment with medication (typically SSRIs) for children with an anxiety disorder, CBT has typically been used as the first line of treatment before initiating a trial of medication. The Child/Adolescent Anxiety Multimodal (CAM) trial compared CBT, SSRI, CBT, and SSRI, and placebo for treatment of anxiety disorders in children aged 7–17-yearsold (Walkup et al., 2008; Rapee et al., 2023). Initial results appeared to reveal a benefit from the combined treatment. Although examination of longer term outcomes revealed less differences among the treatment groups, it was also reported that the acute positive response to treatment may have decreased the risk for chronic anxiety (Ginsburg et al., 2018).

Parent Training

There is variability in the literature regarding the efficacy of adding parent training to treatment of childhood anxiety disorders. Some analyses did not find a difference in outcomes when parent training was added to treatment protocols vs. no parent training (James et al., 2020; Reynolds et al., 2012). However, it is notable that there was reported to be great variability in the type and extent of parent training in the studies included in these reviews (Rapee et al., 2023). Moreover, in an analysis completed by Manassis and colleagues (Manassis et al., 2014), it was reported that anxiety management training for parents resulted in greater maintenance of treatment.

"Virtual/Online" Services

The use of remote medical and psychological services via digital technology increased sharply during the COVID-19 pandemic, and this type of care has continued to be offered by some providers. Results of a recent randomized controlled trial of online support and intervention for child anxiety completed by Cresswell and colleagues revealed a similar reduction in anxiety and improvements in daily functioning for children participating in a parent-led CBT-type of therapy taught online compared to children who received the standard CBT (Creswell et al., 2024).

AUTHORS' COMMENTARY

Online/digital "telemedicine" services have opened up many new possibilities for helping children and their families. They have helped address challenges such as transportation difficulties and distance from the provider. However, providers need to be aware of challenges that can be specifically associated with online care, such as privacy/confidentiality (for example, discussing domestic violence when a perpetrator may be listening in another room).

FUTURE

A child with an anxiety disorder, particularly a disorder that is untreated, is at risk for both academic and social problems at school; problems with friends and future partners; self-harm; and issues with substance misuse (Wehry et al., 2015). In addition to the risk of future problems with anxiety, being diagnosed with an anxiety disorder during childhood increases a person's risk of other mental health disorders in the future, including mood disorders (Costello et al., 2003; Magson et al., 2022; Pine et al., 1998) and eating disorders (Convertino & Blashill, 2022; Hughes, 2012).

CASE STUDIES

Aurora's therapist outside of school collaborated with the speech-language pathologist and counselor at Aurora's school. It was observed that Aurora tended to play with one or two specific children at school, so a game with the three children that included puppets was initiated by the school counselor during free play. Aurora began to speak to the two other children. Aurora continued to work with her therapist and her sessions included a combination of play therapy and CBT. Aurora was enrolled in a summer camp, and one of her friends attended the camp as well. Aurora spoke with her friend at camp, as well as some of the other campers. Toward the end of the summer program, she began answering her camp counselor's questions.

Aurora continued to work with her therapist and she continued to become more comfortable speaking at school during kindergarten and first grade. Although Aurora continued to be considered somewhat shy, there were no additional concerns during the rest of her school years.

Ava began receiving intensive counseling. Initially she did not speak a great deal, but she gradually informed the counselor that she worried all the time that her mother or father would die just like her pet did. She was thinking about her parents all the time and worried that when she was at school, something "bad" would happen to them. Ava was diagnosed with separation anxiety. Cognitive behavioral therapy was initiated. In addition to working with a counselor outside of school, Ava was also scheduled to meet regularly with the school counselor, and with parental permission, both counselors exchanged information regularly. At one point, a referral for a medication consultation was considered, but it was decided to defer this, as Ava's anxiety was gradually decreasing. Ava's school refusal and persistent worries about her parents resolved by the middle of third grade. However, Ava continued to be considered a fairly anxious child, and during high school, Ava began experiencing panic attacks. Ava was diagnosed with a panic disorder and treated with medication.

Final note: Anxiety is a very common symptom and also a relatively common mental health diagnosis. Helping children learn to manage and cope with anxiety provoking situations will provide an important contribution to their "life skills tool kit." Being diagnosed with a specific anxiety disorder increases a child's risk of other anxiety disorders and other mental health diagnoses, particularly if it is left untreated.

HANDOUT FOR CAREGIVERS

Anxiety

Feelings of worry, anxiety, and fearfulness are experienced by everyone, including children. In addition, worrying about your child is part of being a parent. But sometimes the amount of worrying exhibited by your child may appear excessive and concerning. An anxiety disorder is characterized by an intense amount of fear and anxiety that has a negative impact on a person's functioning.

If a Parent Has a History of Anxiety, Does This Increase the Child's Risk of Anxiety?
Having a parent with anxiety, as well as some other mental health diagnoses, can increase a child's risk of also experiencing anxiety. Regardless of the cause, the most important thing is to seek professional help in order for your child to learn to recognize the "triggers" for their worrying and learn techniques to gain control over, and decrease, their anxiety.

Some Techniques to Assist All Children Manage Anxiety

It is important to acknowledge a child's fear/anxiety. Let them know that you understand that their feelings are valid. Provide them with comfort and reassurance that their loved ones will always do their best to protect them.

Gradually help a child become desensitized to anxiety provoking issues (this is a technique that is included in cognitive behavioral therapy [CBT]). For example, if a child is fearful of insects, create stories about insects and encourage them to draw pictures of insects; have them view an insect outside at a comfortable distance and very gradually decrease their distance from the insect as tolerated. Help the child "gain control" over their fears, rather than their fears controlling them.

Create a routine for separation from young children – not too long or too intense a routine, as you want to avoid increasing the child's anxiety. For example, read a story together about going to daycare that involves a "special" good-bye routine – a special ("secret") hug, handshake, or phrase – then together create your own good-bye routine.

Behavioral Therapy

Behavioral therapy is typically the first line of treatment for children with anxiety disorders. Collaboration between the child's family members, therapists, and school staff is an important part of their therapy program. Behavioral therapy often involves CBT, but depending on the age and specific diagnosis of the child, play therapy and/or other therapies might also be recommended. Medications can also be used to treat anxiety, although should be used with caution in children and require close medical follow-up.

BIBLIOGRAPHY

Achenbach T.M., & Rescorla L.A. (2001). Manual for the ASEBE school-age forms & profiles: An integrated system of multi-informant assessment. *Achenbach System of Empirically Based Assessment. Child Behavior Checklist (CBCL)*. Burlington, Vermont: University of Vermont, Research Center from Children, Youth, & Families.

Anxiety Disorders Association of America. www.adaa.org.

Anxiety and Depression Association of America. https://adaa.org.

American Psychiatric Association (APA) (2013). *Diagnostic and Statistical Manual of Mental Disorders – 5th edition*. Arlington, VA: American Psychiatric Association Publishing.

Association for Behavioral and Cognitive Therapies. www.abct.org.

Birmaher B., Khetarpal S., Brent D., Cully M., McKenzie S., Balach L., Kaufman J., & Neer S.M. (1997). The screen for child anxiety related disorders (SCARED): Scale construction and psychometric characteristics. *Journal of the American Academy of Child and Adolescent Psychiatry*, 36:4 545–553. https://doi.org/10.1097/00004583-199704000-00018.

The Child Anxiety Network. www.childanxiety.net.

Convertino, A. D., & Blashill, A. J. (2022). Psychiatric comorbidity of eating disorders in children between the ages of 9 and 10. *Journal of Child Psychology and Psychiatry*, 63 (5): 519–526. https://doi.org/10.1111/jcpp.13484. Epub 2021 Jul 5.

Costello, E., Mustillo, S., Erkanli, A., Keeler, G., & Angold, A. (2003). Prevalence and development of psychiatric disorders in childhood and adolescence. *Archives of General Psychiatry*, 60 (8): 837–844. https://doi.org/10.1001/archpsyc.60.8.837.

Creswell, C., Taylor, L., Giles, S., Howitt, S., Radley, L., Whitaker, E., Brooks, E., Knight, F., Ray, V., van Santen, J., Williams, N., Mort, S., Harris, V., Yu, S., Pollard, J., Violato, M., Waite, P., & Yu, L-M (2024). Digitally augmented, parent-led CBT versus treatment as usual for child anxiety problems in child mental health services in England and Northern Ireland: A pragmatic, non-inferiority, clinical effectiveness and cost-effectiveness randomized controlled trial. *Lancet Psychiatry*, 11: 193–209. doi:10.1016/S2215-0366(23)00429-7. Epub 2024 Feb 6.

Cummings, C. M., Caporino, N., & Kendall, P.C. (2014). Comorbidity of anxiety and depression in children and adolescents: 20 years after. *Psychological Bulletin*, 140 (3): 816–845. https://doi.org/10.1037/a0034733. Epub 2013 Nov 11.

Dickson, S. J., Kuhnert, R.-L., Lavell, C. H., & Rapee, R. M. (2022). Impact of psychotherapy for children and adolescents with anxiety disorders on global and domain-specific functioning: A systematic review and meta-analysis. *Clinical Child and Family Psychology Review,* 25 (4): 720–736. https://doi.org/10.1007/s10567-022-00402-7. Epub 2022 Jul 7.

Evans, R., Clark, D. M., & Leigh, E. (2021). Are young people with primary social anxiety disorder less likely to recover following generic CBT compared to young people with other primary anxiety disorders? A systematic review and meta-analysis. *Behavioural and Cognitive Psychotherapy,* 49(3): 352–369. https://doi.org/10.1017/S135246582000079x. Epub 2020 Dec 10.

Fox, N. A., Snidman, N., Haas, S. A., Degnan, K. A., & Kagan, J. (2015). The relation between infant reactivity at 4 months and behavioral inhibition in the second year. *Infancy,* 20: 98–114. https://doi.org/10.1111/infa.12063.

Garber, S. W., Garber, M. D., & Spizman, R. F. (1993) *Monsters Under the Bed and Other Childhood Fears: Helping Your Child Overcome Anxieties, Fears, and Phobias.* New York City, NY: Villard Books.

Ginsburg, G. S., Becker-Haimes, E. M., Keeton, C., Kendall, P. C., Iyengar, S., Sakolsky, D., Albano, A. M., Peris, T., Compton, S. N., & Piacentini, J. (2018). Results from the child/adolescent anxiety multimodal extended long-term study (CAMELS): Primary anxiety outcomes. *Journal of the American Academy of Child & Adolescent Psychiatry,* 57(7): 471–480. doi: 10.1016/j.jaac.2018.03.017. Epub 2018 May 9.

Hughes, E. K. (2012). Comorbid depression and anxiety in childhood and adolescent anorexia nervosa: Prevalence and implications for outcome. *Clinical Psychologist,* 16(1): 15–24. https://doi.org/10.1111/j.1742-9552.2011.00034.x.

Hussain, F. S., Dobson, E. T., & Strawn, J. R. (2016). Pharmacologic treatment of pediatric anxiety disorders. *Current Treatment Options in Psychiatry,* 3(2): 151–160. https://doi.org/10.1007/s40501-016-0076-7.

James, A. C., Reardon, T., Soler, A., James, G., & Creswell, C. (2020). Cognitive behavioural therapy for anxiety disorders in children and adolescents. *Cochrane Database of Systematic Reviews,* 11(11): CD013162. https://doi.org/10.1002/14651858.

Kagan, J., Reznick, J. S., Clarke, C., Snidman, N., & Garcia-Coll, C. (1984). Behavioral inhibition to the unfamiliar. *Child Development,* 55: 2212–2225.

Kagan, J., Snidman, N., & Arcus, D. (1998). Childhood derivatives of high and low reactivity in infancy. *Child Development,* 69(6): 1483–1493.

Khanal, P., Ståhlberg, T., Luntamo, T., Gyllenberg, D., Kronström, K., Suominen, A., & Soutander, A. (2022). Time trends in treated incidence, sociodemographic risk factors and comorbidities: A Finnish nationwide study on anxiety disorders. *BMC Psychiatry*, 22(1): 144. https://doi.org/10.1186/s12888-022-03743-3.

Lai, M.-C., Kassee, C., Besney, R., Bonata, S., Hull, L., Mandy, W., Szatmari, P., & Ameis, S. H. (2019). Prevalence of co-occurring mental health diagnoses in the autism population: A systematic review and meta-analysis. *The Lancet Psychiatry*, 6 (10): 819–829. https://doi.org/10.1016/S2215-0366(19)30289-5. Epub 2019 Aug 22.

Lawrence, P. J., Murayama, K., & Creswell, C. (2019). Systematic review and meta-analysis: Anxiety and depressive disorders in offspring of parents with anxiety disorders. *Journal of the American Academy of Child & Adolescent Psychiatry*, 58(1): 46–60. https://doi.org/10.1016/j.jaac.2018.07.898. Epub 2018 Nov 1.

Lee, P. H., Feng, Y. A., & Smoller, J. W. (2021). Pleiotropy and cross-disorder genetics among psychiatric disorders. *Biological Psychiatry*, 89 (1): 20–31. https://doi.org/10.1016/j.biopsych.2020.09.026. Epub 2020 Oct 10.

Liu, R., & Bell, M. A. (2020). Fearful temperament and the risk for child and adolescent anxiety: The role of attention biases and effortful control. *Clinical Child and Family Psychology Review*, 23(2): 205–228. doi: 10.1007/s10567-019-00306-z.

Magson, N. R., van Zalk, N., Mörtberg, E., Chard, I., Tillfors, M., & Rapee, R. M., (2022). Latent stability and change in subgroups of social anxiety and depressive symptoms in adolescence: A latent profile and transitional analysis. *Journal of Anxiety Disorders*, Apr (87): 102537. doi: 10.1016/j.janxdis.2022.102537. Epub 2022 Jan 31.

Manassis, K., Lee, T. C., Bennett, K., Zhao, X. Y., Mendlowitz, S., Duda, S., Saini, M., Wilansky, P., Baer, S., Barrett, P., Bodden, D., Cobham, V. E., Dadds, M. R., Flannery-Schroeder, E., Ginsburg, G., Heyne, D., Hudson, J. L., Kendall P. C., Liber, J., Masia-Warner, C., Nauta, M. H., Rappe, R. M., Silverman, W., Siqueland, L., Spence, S. H., Utens, E., & Wood, J. J. (2014). Types of parental involvement in CBT with anxious youth: A preliminary meta-analysis. *Journal of Consulting and Clinical Psychology*, 82 (6): 1163–1172. https://doi.org/10.1037/a0036969. Epub 2014 May 19.

March J. S., Parker J. D. A., Sullivan K., Stallings P., & Conners C. K. (1997). The multidimensional anxiety scale for children (MASC): Factor, structure, reliability, and validity. *Journal of the American Academy of Child & Adolescent Psychiatry*, 36(4): 554–565. https://doi.org/10.1097/00004583-199704000-00019.

Morrison, J. (2014). *DSM-5 Made Easy. The Clinician's Guide to Diagnosis.* New York, NY: The Guilford Press.

Penninx, B. W., Pine, D. S., Holmes, E. A., & Reif, A. (2021). Anxiety disorders. *Lancet*, 397(10277): 914–927. doi: 10.1016/S0140-6736(21)00359-7. Epub 2021 Feb 11.

Pine, D. S., Cohen, P., Gurley, D., Brook, J., & Ma, Y. (1998). The risk for early-adulthood anxiety and depressive disorders in adolescents with anxiety and depressive disorders. *Archives of General Psychiatry*, 55: 56–64. https://doi.org/10.1001/archpsyc.55.1.56.

Rapee, R. M., & Coplan, R. J. (2010). Conceptual relations between anxiety disorder and fearful temperament. In H. Gazelle & K. H. Rubin (Eds.), *Social Anxiety in Childhood: Bridging Developmental and Clinical Perspectives, New Directions for Child and Adolescent Development*, Vol. 127 (pp. 17–31). San Francisco: Jossey-Bass.

Rapee, R. M., Creswell, C., Kendall, P. C., Pine, D. S., & Waters, A. M. (2023). Anxiety disorders in children and adolescents: A summary and overview of the literature. *Behaviour Research and Therapy*, 168: 104376. https://doi.org/10.1016/j.brat.2023.104376. Epub 2023 Jul 20.

Rapee, R. M., Lyneham, H. J., Hudson, J. L., Kangas, M., Wuthrich, V. M., & Schniering, C. A. (2013). The effect of comorbidity on treatment of anxious children and adolescents: Results from a large, combined sample. *Journal of the American Academy of Child & Adolescent Psychiatry*, 52 (1): 47–56. https://doi.org/10.1016/j.jaac.2012.10.002. Epub 2012 Dec 1.

Rapee, R. M., Magson, N. R., Forbes, M. K., Richardson, C. E., Johnco, C. J., Oar, E. L., & Fardouly, J. (2022b). Risk for social anxiety in early adolescence: Longitudinal impact of pubertal development, appearance comparisons, and peer connections. *Behaviour Research and Therapy*, 154: 104126. https://doi.org/10.1016/j.brat.2022.104126. Epub 2022 May 20,

Rapee, R. M., McLellan, L. F., Carl, T., Trompeter, N., Hudson, J. L., Jones, M.P., & Wuthrick, V. M. (2022a). Comparison of transdiagnostic treatment and specialized social anxiety treatment for children and adolescents with social anxiety disorder: A randomized controlled trial. *Journal of the American Academy of Child & Adolescent Psychiatry*, 62(6): 646–655. https://doi.org/10.1016/j.jaac.2022.08.003. Epub 2022 Aug 17.

Rapee, R. M., Schniering, C. A., & Hudson, J. L. (2009). Anxiety disorders during childhood and adolescence: Origins and treatment. *Annual Review of Clinical Psychology*, 5: 311–341.

Reynolds, S., Wilson, C., Austin, J., & Hooper, L. (2012). Effects of psychotherapy for anxiety in children and adolescents: A meta-analytic review. *Clinical Psychology Review*, 32 (4): 251–262.

Riddle M. A., Ginsberg G. S., Walkup J. T., Labelarte M. J., Pine D. S., Davies M., Greenhill, L., Sweeney, M., Klein, R., Abikoff, H., Hack, S., Klee, B., McCracken, J., Bergman, L., Piacentini, J., March, J., Compton, S., Robinson, J., O'Hara, T., Roper, M., & Research Units on Pediatric Psychopharmacology Anxiety Study Group (2002). The pediatric anxiety rating scale (PARS): Development and psychometric properties. *Journal of the American Academy of Child & Adolescent Psychiatry*, 42(9): 1061–1069. https://doi.org/10.1097/00004583-200209000-00006.

Strawn J. R., Dobson E. T., & Giles L. L. (2017). Primary pediatric care psychopharmacology: Focus on medications for ADHD, depression and anxiety. *Current Problems in Pediatric & Adolescent Health Care*, 47(1): 3–14. https://doi.org/10.1016/j.cppeds.2016.11.008. Epub 2016 Dec 30.

Strawn, J. R., Lu, L., Peris, T. S., Levine, A., & Walkup, J. T. (2021). Research Review: Pediatric anxiety disorders – what have we learnt in the last 10 years? *Journal of Child Psychology and Psychiatry*, 62(2):114–139. https://doi.org/10.1111/jcpp.13262. Epub 2020 Jun 5.

Vicente, B., Saldivia, S., de la Barra, F., Kohn, R., Pihan, R., Valdivia, M., Rioseco, P., & Melipillan, R. (2012). Prevalence of child and adolescent mental disorders in Chile: A community epidemiological study. *Journal of Child Psychology and Psychiatry*, 53(10): 1026–1035. https://doi.org/10.1111/j.1469-7610.2012.02566.x. Epub 2012 May 31.

Walkup, J. T., Albano, A. M., Piacentini, J., Birmaher, B., Compton, S.N., Sherrill, J. T., Ginsburg, G. S., Rynn, M. A., McCracken, J., Waslick, B., Iyengar, S., March, J. S., & Kendall, P. C. (2008). Cognitive behavioral therapy, sertraline, or a combination in childhood anxiety. *New England Journal of Medicine*, 359(26): 2753–2766. https://doi.org/10.1056/NEJMoa0804633. Epub 2008 Oct 30.

Wang, Z., Whiteside, S. P. H., Sim, L., Farrah, W., Morrow, A. S., Alsawas, M., Barrionuevo, P., Tello, M., Asi, N., Beuschel, B., Daraz, L., Almasri, J., Zaiem, F., Larrea-Mantilla, L., Ponce, O. J., LeBlanc, A., Prokop, L. J., & Murad, M.H. (2017). Comparative effectiveness and safety of cognitive behavioral therapy and pharmacotherapy for childhood anxiety disorders: A systematic review and meta-analysis. *Journal of the American Medical Association (JAMA) – Pediatrics*. 171(11): 1049–1056. https://doi.org/10.1001/jamapediatrics.2017.3036.

Waszczuk, M. A., Zavos, H. M., Gregory, A.M., & Eley, T. C. (2014). The phenotypic and genetic structure of depression and anxiety disorder symptoms in childhood, adolescence, and young adulthood, *Journal of the American Medical Association – Psychiatry*, 71(8): 905–916. https://doi.org/10.1001/jamapsychiatry.2014.655.

Wehry A. M., Beesdo-Baum, K., Hennelly, M. M., Connolly, S. D., & Strawn, J. R. (2015). Assessment and treatment of anxiety disorders in children and adolescents. *Current Psychiatry Reports*, 17(7): 591. https://doi.org/10.1007/s11920-015-0591-z.

Wilson, R. & Lyons, L. (2013). *Anxious Kids Anxious Parents. 7 Ways to Stop the Worry Cycle and Raise Courageous & Independent Children*. Deerfield Beach, FL: Health Communications, Inc.

Worry Wise Kids. www.worrywisekids.org.

CHAPTER 9

Depression or Just Moody?

L et us discuss three children who each present with the same story.

CASE STUDIES

Harper, **Leo**, and **Mia** are each 11 years old and attending fifth grade. Each of them has always been considered a good student, but this year their academic performance has not been optimal. Initially it was felt that their moodiness and poor school performance were related to them entering the "tween" years, but recently their parents and teachers have been concerned. The parents of all three children gave permission for their children to meet with the school counselor.

TEMPERAMENT VS. MOOD

Temperament includes behavioral traits – for example, a child may be described as "rigid," "irritable," "easygoing," "difficult," or "high strung." Mood is an affective state that can change based on an individual's circumstances – for example, anxious, sad, or happy. Depression, also known as major depressive disorder or clinical depression, is a type of mood disorder.

DEPRESSION

Everyone experiences a range of emotions, including periods of sadness. Sadness can affect a child's sleep patterns, their appetite, and their

DOI: 10.4324/9781003639121-9

relationships with their family and peers. But when is a child's sadness a concern for depression? Depression is a type of mood disorder. In addition to clinical depression/major depressive disorder, there are other "types" of depressive disorders – for example, dysthymic disorder; depression related to a medical condition, a medication or menstruation; and disruptive mood dysregulation disorder (American Psychiatric Association, 2013 [APA]; Morrison 2014). The diagnosis of depression in this chapter will be used to refer to clinical depression or major depressive disorder unless otherwise specified.

Although depression is more common in adolescents, younger children can also present with symptoms of this diagnosis. Symptoms of childhood depression can include feelings of sadness, irritability, self-injurious behaviors, and/or a change in appetite and/or sleep patterns (APA, 2013; Morrison, 2014).

Depression is a clinical diagnosis based on a thorough history and psychological assessment. A child's presentation and information from the child, family members, teachers, and other school professionals are important when making this diagnosis. Diagnosing depression can sometimes be challenging, as some children may not talk about their feelings; they may not necessarily appear sad, as their depression may result in misbehavior or the appearance of poor motivation; they may also appear anxious, and it is not unusual for anxiety and depression to occur together. Some children may complain of physical discomfort – for example, headaches and abdominal discomfort. There are questionnaires that can be helpful in screening for depressive disorders – for example, Beck Depression Inventory (Beck et al., 1988); Children's Depression Inventory (Kovacs, 1981; Saylor et al., 1984); Center for Epidemiological Studies Depression Scale for Children (CAS-DC) (Roberts et al., 1990); and Severity Measure for Depression—Child Age 11–17 (PHQ-A) (Calonge et al., 2009).

PREVALENCE

Similar to other mental health diagnoses, a range of prevalence of childhood depression has been reported. Results of a meta-analysis of 41 studies examining the reported prevalence of childhood depressive disorders from 2004 to 2019 in children less than 13 years old revealed a pooled total prevalence of 1.07%, with estimates of 0.71% for major depressive disorder, 0.30% for dysthymia, and 1.6% for disruptive mood dysregulation disorder. The estimates showed no significant difference with respect to gender or income (Spoelma et al., 2023). Gender differences, however, have been consistently reported after puberty, with girls being more likely to experience depression by age 15. There have also been recent studies that reported an increase in depressive symptoms in children associated with the COVID-19 pandemic (Bignardi et al., 2020; Larsen et al., 2023).

CASE STUDIES

Before **Harper** met with the school counselor, her parents felt that the counselor should be aware that their family had been undergoing some stress, and that they were seeing a marriage counselor. Harper met with the school counselor, and she informed the counselor that her parents' frequent arguing was upsetting to her.

Leo's parents reported that Leo had been struggling with his schoolwork that year. Leo informed the school counselor that he felt he was "stupid." Leo's parents reported that throughout elementary school Leo had worked very hard, putting maximum effort into his schoolwork. Even though several of Leo's teachers had expressed some concerns about his academic performance, he was able to pass each grade. In addition, because Leo's teachers felt that Leo had difficulty paying attention in school, Leo had been treated with psychostimulant medication since third grade.

Mia met with the counselor at school. Initially her interaction was limited. However, she did report that she had not been sleeping well and that she rarely ate lunch at school. When asked about peers, she did not engage in eye contact and shrugged her shoulders.

CAUSES OF DEPRESSION

Similar to anxiety, a family history of depression or other mental health diagnoses, can increase a child's risk for this diagnosis. In addition, stressful life events and family challenges can be precursors to depression – for example, trauma, stress, maltreatment, bullying, and social rejection.

A child's sadness in response to stressful life events does not always develop into a diagnosis of depression. However a child with a history of trauma should be monitored for symptoms of depression, as well as other emotional disorders.

There is no lab test or neuroimaging study that can definitively confirm or rule out depression. Research studies have attempted to explore neurological differences that may exist in individuals who may be more prone to mental health diagnoses, including depression. For example, Luking and colleagues completed functional magnetic resonance (MRI) imaging studies in a group of 7-to 11-year-old children with a history of major depressive disorder or a maternal history of depression, and results revealed some anomalies in the relationship between the amygdala and some of the regions of cognitive control (Luking et al., 2011).

THE COVID-19 PANDEMIC

The psychological, physical, and social impact of the COVID-19 pandemic warrants an entire book. But we feel that it is worth briefly discussing this major event as part of this chapter. It seems logical that school closures, virtual instruction, and limited social interaction with peers would have an impact on children's mental health, and some research has confirmed this. Bignardi and colleagues completed mental health assessments of 168 children in the UK, aged 7.6–11.6 years, 18 months before and also during the UK lockdown using the Revised Child Anxiety and Depression Scales (RCADS) short form. Results revealed a statistically significant increase in depressive symptoms, with no difference across demographic groups, including age, gender, and family socioeconomic status (Bignardi et al., 2020). A study completed in China assessed rates of depression and anxiety in adolescents during the COVID-19 pandemic and reported an increase in anxiety and depression, with being female and in the senior year of high school associated with an increase in symptoms. It is also interesting to note that they found that a sleep duration of at least six hours and exercising at least 30 minutes per day were associated with a decrease in symptoms (Chen et al., 2021). In Norway, Larsen and colleagues found an increase in internalizing symptoms in children later in the pandemic. Symptoms of anxiety did not increase during the initial lockdown in March 2020 but increased during the second lockdown. They also found that depressive symptoms increased after the social distancing protocols were gradually removed, which they hypothesized may be due to the "sleeper effect", i.e., a delayed effect of the protocol; a response to the challenges of going back to school; or a reflection of the difficulty of re-establishing the family's previous routine. This increase in depressive symptoms associated with the gradual elimination of lockdown was found to be more significant in younger children, and the impact of the pandemic was stronger in children who had preexisting mental health challenges (Larsen et al., 2023).

AUTHORS' COMMENTARY

Studying the psychological effects of the COVID-19 pandemic on children and adolescents will be an ongoing process. Understanding the emotional toll on children and their families will assist in planning ways to lessen the negative effects of future global traumatic events.

OTHER DIAGNOSES THAT CAN PRESENT WITH SYMPTOMS OF DEPRESSION (OR OCCUR CO-MORBIDLY WITH DEPRESSION)

The initial presentation of childhood depression may be behavioral problems at school and/or at home, irritability, lack of energy/tiredness, a change in sleep patterns, and loss of interest in previously preferred activities. These symptoms are shared with other diagnoses, including the following.

Anxiety

As described in Chapter 8, symptoms of depression can overlap with symptoms of anxiety in children. In addition, it is not uncommon for a diagnosis of depression to occur co-morbidly with an anxiety disorder, especially in adolescents.

Attention-Deficit/Hyperactivity Disorder (ADHD)

Presenting symptoms of ADHD often include poor attention, tense/restlessness, anxiety, and sleep problems, and sometimes learning/school difficulties – these can also be symptoms of depression. In addition, suboptimal self-esteem can be observed in children who have been diagnosed with various social-emotional challenges, including the diagnoses of both ADHD and depression.

Physical Illnesses

Some physical illnesses can be associated with symptoms that overlap with depressive symptoms – for example, thyroid dysfunction, anemia, diabetes, and some infectious diseases such as Epstein–Bar virus/mononucleosis.

Prolonged Grief Disorder

This was a new diagnosis added to the 2022 revised *Diagnostic and Statistical Manual of Mental Disorders – 5th edition* (DSM-5-TR). Grief is a natural response after the death of a loved one. However, this diagnosis is given when the response to the death of a loved one is more severe, intense, and prolonged than what is considered typical. This diagnosis is more specific than clinical depression as it is directly related to the loss of the child's loved one (American Psychiatric Association [APA], 2022).

Trauma-Related Disorders, Including Posttraumatic Stress Disorder (PTSD)

This can present with some symptoms that overlap with the diagnosis of depression. This diagnosis is discussed in Chapter 11.

AUTHORS' COMMENTARY

We feel that it is worth repeating that when a child is given a mental health diagnosis, this often increases the child's risk for other mental health diagnoses – for example, a child who is diagnosed with anxiety is at an increased risk for depression, and vice versa. Children who are diagnosed with depression are also at an increased risk for school failure, social difficulties, and self-harm.

CASE STUDIES

The counselor recommended that **Harper** and her parents begin family counseling. Through counseling, Harper was able to gradually express her feelings. She was concerned that she may be the cause of her parents' disagreements. Harper was provided with reassurance about her role within her family and both of her parents' unconditional love for her.

Leo's fifth-grade teacher confirmed that Leo was having academic difficulty in school. It was requested that a multidisciplinary team evaluation be completed.

Mia began meeting regularly with the counselor both individually and as part of a social lunch group. During the lunch group, another student mentioned that there were some girls at school who were "mean" to Mia. Mia became teary eyed.

AUTHOR'S COMMENTARY

Bullying can threaten a child's safety and their physical and emotional well-being, and have a negative impact on their ability to learn. Bullying has become a popular topic of conversation. Did bullying always exist? The answer is yes; but the internet and social media have added a new and dangerous layer to childhood (and adult) bullying. Children who are the victim of bullying are at an increased risk for mental health challenges including symptoms of anxiety and depression.

As adults, we should consistently send the message that bullying is unacceptable behavior. Although bullying may never be completely extinguished, it is important to talk about the effects of this issue and create communities and schools where bullying is treated seriously. It is also important to be proactive by training both students and school staff to prevent bullying and address it immediately. In addition to formal school programs, teaching children about bullying can include writing and other creative arts programs.

CASE STUDIES

Although **Harper's** parents separated for a period of time, Harper continued to participate in counseling and her mood improved. She enjoyed participating in music-related activities and both of her parents remained actively involved in her life.

Results of **Leo's** public school multidisciplinary evaluation revealed an average IQ but some academic scores below grade and age expectations. Leo was diagnosed with a learning disability. It was also noted that Leo had difficulty processing information, and further evaluation confirmed the diagnosis of an auditory processing disorder. An individualized education program (IEP) was created, and Leo's academic performance and mood gradually improved.

Mia began meeting with a counselor outside of school. She eventually confirmed being the victim of bullying and shared with her counselor some of the cruel comments made about her on social media. She disclosed that the bullying had been going on for at least two years. She expressed that she felt that her life was horrible; she had found some relief from her emotional pain by cutting herself. The diagnosis of depression was confirmed, and Mia began working intensively with a psychologist and was also referred for a psychiatric consultation.

TREATMENT

A healthy, positive lifestyle is always a goal for children, including an appropriate amount of sleep, a variety of healthy foods in their diet, opportunities for physical exercise, and supportive school and home environments. Although a goal, a healthy lifestyle unfortunately will not necessarily prevent or fully treat depression. Treatment for depression involves counseling and therapy. In addition to treatment of anxiety, cognitive behavioral therapy (CBT) is often used to treat depression. Cognitive behavioral therapy provides children with tools to cope with their emotions and change negative thoughts into more positive, productive thoughts and activities. Family therapy can also be beneficial. Often a combination of CBT and family therapy may be needed.

The "first line" of medication to treat depression is often selective serotonin reuptake inhibitors (SSRI). These medications increase the level of serotonin in the brain, as serotonin increases feelings of well-being and happiness. Although some SSRI medications have been approved for use in elementary-school-aged children who have been diagnosed with depression, they must be used with caution and with close medical follow-up (Strawn et al., 2017).

There have been multiple studies completed regarding the efficacy of treatment with medication, psychological interventions, or both, in treatment of depression in children and adolescents. Results of a 2020 meta-analysis of 71 trials of treatments for depression reported that, despite a somewhat limited amount of "high-quality evidence", fluoxetine (an SSRI) alone or in combination with CBT appeared to be the most efficacious acute treatment of moderate-to-severe depressive disorder in children and adolescents. The authors also added that there was variability in response to treatments and interventions, so "clinicians should carefully balance the risk-benefit profile of efficacy, acceptability, and suicide risk of all active interventions in young patients with depression on a case-by-case basis" (Zhou et al., 2020). In another 2020 review of studies assessing treatments for depression, it was reported that in adolescents with major depressive disorder, CBT, fluoxetine, escitalopram (another SSRI), and combined fluoxetine and CBT appear to improve depressive symptoms. However, it was also reported that treatment with SSRIs was sometimes reported to be associated with adverse effects in adolescents or children with major depressive disorder. No harm from psychotherapy was reported (Viswanathan et al., 2020). It should be added that in 2004 the U.S. Food and Drug Administration (FDA) placed a black warning label on antidepressant medications, warning that antidepressants can increase the risk of suicidal thinking and behavior in children and adolescents with major depression and other psychiatric disorders. It is important for all parents to review all risks with their child's prescribing physician.

WHAT CAN BE DONE ABOUT A CHILD'S FEELINGS OF SADNESS, EVEN IF IT IS NOT FELT THAT THE CHILD IS CLINICALLY DEPRESSED?

Sadness is a normal emotion and is experienced by all children. As previously stated, a healthy, positive lifestyle is always a goal for children, including an appropriate amount of sleep, a variety of healthy foods in their diet, opportunities for physical exercise, and supportive school and home environments. When a child is sad, irritable, or expressing other negative emotions, it is important to listen to them and acknowledge their feelings. Explore with the child the activities they enjoy and that make them feel happy and relaxed. Attempt to assist in transitioning their negative feelings into more positive thoughts and actions. Even if a child is not felt to be clinically depressed, working with a therapist or counselor may be helpful in order for them to begin to understand their feelings and emotions and develop coping skills.

SUICIDE RISK

Depression can result in a child thinking about, planning, or attempting to harm themselves. If a child endorses thoughts of self-harm or states negative comments such as, "I wish I was dead," it can sometimes be challenging to determine whether these statements are stated out of anger, a "dramatic effect," an impulsive statement, or true suicidal ideation. Of course, it is always appropriate to request further assessment with a professional who has expertise in this area – for example, the local Crisis Center or emergency department. A child who has a plan for self-harm or who actually makes a suicide attempt requires an emergency assessment and treatment.

CASE STUDIES

Mia received intensive counseling. Although antibullying programs were implemented at school, and addressed cyberbullying, Mia continued to present with a negative mood. Mia expressed suicidal ideation and was referred to a psychiatrist. She was started on treatment with an SSRI medication and continued to receive intensive counseling that included CBT and family therapy. Mia's mood gradually improved, and she began to show more interest in socializing with her close friends. The staff at school were aware of the history of bullying. Mia was very gradually weaned off SSRI medication in seventh grade. She continued to receive psychiatric follow-up throughout high school and college and required treatment with medication again as a young adult.

HANDOUT FOR CAREGIVERS

Depressive Disorders

All children experience a range of emotions and moods, including periods of sadness. Sadness can affect a child's sleep patterns, their appetite, and their relationships with their family and peers. But when is a child's sadness a concern for depression? Depression is a type of mood disorder. Childhood depression is characterized by severe and prolonged sadness that can have various presentations.

If you have any concerns about your child's sadness or irritability, it is important for you to discuss these with your child's primary care physician who may refer your child for further evaluation with a mental health clinician. **If you are concerned your child might harm themself or others, call your child's mental health practitioner, primary care doctor, or 911 immediately. It is very important that you take any suicidal signs seriously.**

Treatment for childhood depression includes therapy with a clinician who has expertise in working with children with emotional challenges. The therapist should also work collaboratively with other people involved with your child's life, including family members and teachers. If your child's depression is very severe or does not make the appropriate improvement with therapy, a trial of treatment with medication may be considered.

BIBLIOGRAPHY

American Academy of Child & Adolescent Psychiatry – Depression Resource Center. www.aacap.org.

American Psychiatric Association (APA) (2013). *Diagnostic and Statistical Manual of Mental Disorders – 5th edition*. Arlington, VA: American Psychiatric Association Publishing.

American Psychiatric Association (APA) (2022). *Diagnostic and Statistical Manual of Mental Disorders – 5th edition. Text Revision (DSM-5-TR)*. Arlington, VA: American Psychiatric Association Publishing.

Anxiety and Depression Association of America. https://adaa.org.

Beck, A. T., Steer, R. A., & Garbin, M. G. (1988). Psychometric properties of the Beck Depression Inventory: Twenty-five years of evaluation. *Clinical Psychology Review*, 8(1): 77–100. https://doi.org/10.1016/0272-7358(88)90050-5.

Bignardi, G., Dalmaijer, E. S., Anwyl-Irvine, A. L., Smith, T. A., Siugzdaite, R., Uh, S., & Astle, D. E. (2020). Longitudinal increases in childhood depression symptoms during the COVID-19 lockdown. *Archives of Diseases in Children*,106(8): 791–797. https://doi.org/10.1136/archdischild-2020-320372.

Bitsko, R. H., Holbrook, J. R., Ghandour, R. M., Blumberg, S. G., Visser, S. N., Perou, R., & Walkup, J. T. (2018). Epidemiology and impact of health care provider-diagnosed anxiety and depression among US children. *Journal of Developmental and Behavioral Pediatrics*, 39(5): 395–403. https://doi.org/10.1097/DBP.0000000000000571.

Chen, X., Qi, H., Liu, R., Feng, Y., Li, W., Xiang, M., Cheung, T., Jackson, T., Wang, G., & Xiang, Y-T. (2021). Depression, anxiety and associated factors among Chinese adolescents during the COVID-19 outbreak: A comparison of two cross-sectional studies. *Translational Psychiatry*, 11: 148. https://doi.org/10.1038/s41398-021-01271-4.

Kovacs, M. (1981). Rating scales to assess depression in school-aged children. *Acta Paedopsychiatrica: International Journal of Child & Adolescent Psychiatry*, 46(5–6): 305–315.

Larsen, L., Schauber, S. K., Holt, T., & Helland, M. S. (2023). Longitudinal Covid-19 effects on child mental health: Vulnerability and age dependent trajectories. *Child and Adolescent Psychiatry and Mental Health*, 17: 104.

Lima, N. N. R., do Nascimento, V. B., Melo, S., de Carvalho, F., de Abreu, L. C., Neto, M. L. R., Brasil, A. Q., Junior, F. T. C., de Oliveira, G. F., & Reis, A. O. A. (2013). Childhood depression: A systematic review. *Neuropsychiatric Disease and Treatment*, 9: 1417–1425. https://doi.org/10.2147/NDT.S42402.

Luking, K. R., Repovs, G., Belden A. C., Gaffrey, M. S., Botteron, K. N., Luby, J. L., & Barch, D. M. (2011). Functional connectivity of the amygdala in early-childhood-onset depression. *Journal of the American Academy of Child and Adolescent Psychiatry*, 50(10): 1027–1041.e3. https://doi.org/10.1016/j.jaac.2011.07.019. Epub 2011 Sep 3.

Morrison, J. (2014). *DSM-5 Made Easy. The Clinician's Guide to Diagnosis.* New York, NY: The Guilford Press.

Roberts, R. E., Andrews, J. A., Lewinsohn, P. M., & Hops, H. (1990). Assessment of depression in adolescents using the center for epidemiologic studies scale. *Psychological Assessment: A Journal of Consulting and Clinical Psychology*, 2(2), 122–128. https://doi.org/10.1037/1040-3590.2.2.122.

Saylor, C. F., Finch, A. J., & Spirito, A. (1984). The children's depression inventory: A systematic evaluation of psychometric properties. *Journal of Consulting and Clinical Psychology*, 52(6): 955–967. https://doi.org/10.1037//0022-006x.52.6.955.

Siu, A.L., & US Preventive Services Task Force. (2016). Screening for depression in children and adolescents: US preventive services task force recommendation statement. *Pediatrics*, 137(3): e20154467. Epub 2016 Feb 8.

Spoelma, M. J., Sicouri, G. L., Francis, D. A., MclinNeuro, Songco, A. D., Daniel, E. K., & Hudson, J. L. (2023). Estimated prevalence of depressive disorders in children from 2004 to 2019 a systematic review and meta-analysis. *Journal of the American Medical Association Pediatrics*, 177(10): 1017–1027. https://doi.org/10.1001/jamapediatrics.2023.3221.

Strawn, J. R., Dobson, E., & Giles, L (2017). Primary pediatric care psychopharmacology: Focus on medications for ADHD, depression and anxiety. *Current Problems in Pediatric & Adolescent Health Care*, 47(1): 3–14. https://doi.org/10.1016/j.cppeds.2016.11.008. Epub 2016 Dec 30.

Viswanathan, M., Kennedy, S. M., McKeeman, J., Christian, R., Coker-Schwimmer, M., Middleton, J. C., Bann, C., Lux, L., Randolph, C., & Forman-Hoffman, V. (2020). Treatment of depression in children and adolescents: A systematic review. Report No 20-EHC005-EF. *Comparative Effectiveness Review, No. 224.* Department of Health and Human Services www.stopbullying.gov. Rockville, MD: Agency for Healthcare Research and Quality (US).

Zhou, X., Teng, T., Zhang, Y., Del Giovane, C., Furukawa, T. A., Weisa, J. R., Li, X., Cuijpers, P., Coghill, D., Xiang, Y., Hetrick. S. E., Leucht, S., Qui, M., Barth, J., Ravindran, A. V., Yang, L., Curry, J., Fan, L, Silva, S. G., Cipriani, A., & Xie, P. (2020). Comparative efficacy and acceptability of antidepressants, psychotherapies, and their combination for acute treatment of children and adolescents with depressive disorder: A systematic review and network meta-analysis. *Lancet Psychiatry*, 7(7): 591–601. https://doi.org/10.1016/S2215-0366(20)30137-1.

CHAPTER 10

Obsessive-Compulsive Disorder or Just Overly Neat and Clean?

During medical school, students would sometimes hear comments made in an attempt to encourage thorough and meticulous work habits – for example, "Being a little OCD will make you less likely to miss a diagnosis." It is true that being thorough and careful are important qualities that can help one achieve success in many professions. However, behaviors suggestive of an actual diagnosis of obsessive-compulsive disorder (OCD) will interfere with, rather than benefit, an individual's day-to-day functioning.

CASE STUDIES

Sophia is ten years old. Sophia's parents and her fourth grade teacher noticed that Sophia had developed some patches of missing hair on her head, and her eyebrows appeared to be thinning. They had observed her twirling her hair and touching her eyebrows. Her parents started to find clumps of hair on Sophia's bedroom carpet. They asked Sophia's pediatrician to refer her to a dermatologist. However, after unexpectedly entering Sophia's bedroom, they observed that she was pulling hair from her head.

Jack is five years old and was diagnosed with autism spectrum disorder (ASD) when he was two years old. He frequently demonstrates repetitive, stereotypic movements. Jack developed a repetitive behavior of ripping up paper and placing the pieces into the radiator gratings at home. At school Jack's teacher observed Jack demonstrating a similar behavior. Jack's parents inquired whether he may be presenting with OCD in addition to ASD.

DOI: 10.4324/9781003639121-10

When **Levi** was in first grade, he was observed to frequently blink his eyes. The blinking was repetitive and occurred randomly throughout the day – for example, when he was watching TV, completing schoolwork, or even when he was engaged in a preferred activity such as building with toys. He was not bothered by the blinking – in fact, when his parents asked him about the blinking, he reported, "I don't blink, but sometimes my eyebrows burn a little." Levi had an ophthalmology consultation, and no abnormalities were identified. Levi's parents were informed that the eye blinking was likely a simple motor tic. Levi was also observed to have a limited attention span and a high activity level, and he was diagnosed with attention-deficit/hyperactivity disorder (ADHD) during the latter part of first grade. He was started on treatment with a psychostimulant medication at the start of second grade. There was no obvious change in his eye blinking after starting his ADHD medication, and the frequency of his eye blinking continued to be variable. However, towards the middle of second grade, it was observed that Levi was picking at his skin excessively, sometimes resulting in bleeding. In addition to ADHD and tics, his teacher inquired whether Levi may also have an OCD-related disorder?

It is important to first note that some types of intensive and recurrent thoughts and behaviors can be considered developmentally appropriate. Preschool-age children are comforted by certain routines – for example, morning, bedtime, and mealtime routines. These routines provide structure and can be helpful in maintaining family functioning. The concept of "magical thinking" – the idea that one's actions or thoughts can influence or cause unrelated, random external events – is also considered a part of typical early childhood development; a more reality-based principle of causation is acquired as a child matures. School-aged children use rituals and memorization in order to learn group games and activities. Finally, collecting specific items and memorabilia can be an acceptable childhood hobby. These persistent, repetitive types of childhood behaviors can have positive functions – for example, assisting a child in learning to socialize with peers and providing them with structure that can decrease stress. However, if a child's persistent thoughts and ritualistic behaviors become difficult for them to control, result in distress, and interfere with their daily functioning, this can be a cause for concern (Geller et al., 2021).

OCD AND OCD-RELATED DISORDERS

OCD

Obsessions are characterized by very intense, repetitive thoughts and ideas that a person is unable to control. Compulsions are characterized by repetitive behaviors that an individual feels they must do, often related to their obsessions. An individual who is diagnosed with OCD experiences obsessions and compulsions that are intense, excessive, and interfere with their daily functioning. Most individuals who are diagnosed with OCD are aware of, and sometimes even embarrassed about, the problematic nature of their obsessions and compulsions. This can cause them personal distress. Some examples of obsessions and compulsions that can be associated with the diagnosis of OCD include a fear of germs and contamination resulting in frequent, excessive hand washing; doubts about completion of a task that leads to repeatedly checking that the task is done; feeling the need to count or say a specific phrase repetitively before a specific action; a need for "symmetry," which may include counting, repeating, ordering, re-writing; repetitive "unacceptable" thoughts (for example, aggressive, sexual, religious) (American Psychiatric Association [APA], 2013; Morrison, 2014). Childhood OCD indicates an onset before 18 years old, and early onset OCD typically suggests an onset between 6 and 12 years old (Farrell et al., 2023).

OCD-Related Disorders

There are also several OCD-related disorders included in the psychiatric literature, some of which include disorders focused on a person's physical appearance; a compulsion to collect and accumulate things; and pulling out body hair; scratching or picking the skin (APA, 2013; Morrison, 2014).

DIAGNOSIS

The process of evaluating a child for any mental health diagnosis incorporates a thorough history, including a family history; complete physical and neurological examinations; interviews; and psychological/emotional evaluations, often including completion of questionnaires. Ultimately, the diagnosis should be made by a clinician with expertise in childhood mental health disorders. There are several questionnaires – for example, the Children's Yale-Brown Obsessive Compulsive Scale (CY-BOCS) – that can be used to assist in evaluating the severity of obsessions and compulsions when considering a diagnosis of OCD (Scahill, 1997). Adam and colleagues recently presented a systematic review of brief assessment tools that can be used to screen for OCD. Their results revealed evidence that the sensitivity and specificity of the eight-question version of the Child Behavior Checklist-Obsessive Compulsive Subscale (CBCL-OCS) (Nelson et al., 2001) is strong enough to indicate that a referral to a specialist for further evaluation is indicated (Adam et al., 2025).

PREVALENCE

Reports of the prevalence of OCD range from 1% to 4% (Farrell et al., 2023; Nazeer et al., 2020). Over half of adults diagnosed with OCD have been reported to have experienced symptoms as a child. Moreover, onset of OCD during childhood has been reported to be associated with greater severity of symptoms during adolescence and adulthood (Farrell et al., 2023). It is not uncommon for one or more other diagnoses to be present in children with OCD – for example, tic disorder, anxiety disorder, depression, and ADHD. The course of OCD can come and go, but it can also be a chronic condition.

ETIOLOGY

Several possible etiologies for OCD have been studied. Genetics can play a role – for example, there are specific genetic-based disorders that can predispose an individual to various mental health diagnoses, including OCD. In addition, the risk of OCD is greater in first degree relatives of individuals who have been diagnosed with OCD, with an even greater risk if the OCD has a childhood-onset. The concordance rate for monozygotic twins is higher than for dizygotic twins. Other research has explored parenting styles and stressful life events as possible risk factors/triggers. Neuroimaging studies have reported some differences in specific parts of the brain and brain activity, and additional research has pointed to differences in neurotransmitter pathways in individuals with OCD, including the possibility of a deficiency in the neurotransmitter serotonin. Finally, some immunological and infectious precipitants of OCD symptoms have been reported, including pediatric autoimmune neuropsychiatric disorders associated with streptococcal infections (PANDAS) and pediatric acute-onset neuropsychiatric syndrome (PANS) (Nazeer et al., 2020).

AUTHORS' COMMENTARY

Excessive childhood and adolescent screen time has been a "thorn in our side" for much of our careers, so we are naturally intrigued by research in this area. Our bias now revealed, it is interesting to note that in 2022 a prospective study of 9,208 children aged between nine and ten found an association between longer total screen time, particularly playing video games and watching videos, and new-onset OCD at two-year follow-up, even after adjusting for confounding variables and the elimination of children with baseline OCD from the study (Nagata et al., 2022). Although further research is needed in this area, this study supports other research regarding potential risks of excessive screen time in children.

TICS

A tic is a precipitous, involuntary movement or vocalization that is rapid and repetitive, in a random and "non-rhythmical" fashion. Tics are fairly common in school-age children and tend to decrease or even disappear by adolescence. Examples of motor tics include eye-blinking, facial movements (for example, forehead wrinkling), head turning, and shoulder shrugging; examples of vocal tics include throat clearing, sniffling, and coughing, Tics can be precipitated by stress, but they can also occur with no clear precipitant. Tics do not occur during sleep and are more common in boys than in girls.

Although tics are relatively common in children and often resolve spontaneously, in some cases they can persist and become more complicated, transitioning into a chronic motor or vocal tic disorder or sometimes meeting criteria for Tourette syndrome/disorder. A diagnosis of Tourette syndrome requires the presence of motor and vocal tics for an extended period of time. It is also notable that the *Diagnostic and Statistical Manual of Mental Disorders – 5th edition* (DSM-5) includes a specifier for "Tic-related OCD" (APA, 2013; Morrison, 2014).

There is no known single, specific cause of tics, but genetics can play a role. There have also been other factors, including autoimmune conditions, medications, and infections, that have been suggested to sometimes precipitate tics, tic disorders, and Tourette syndrome. Tic disorders and Tourette syndrome are clinical diagnoses. In order to make a diagnosis, a thorough history and examination should be completed.

"HABITS"

The definition of habit includes "an acquired mode of behavior that has become nearly involuntary" (*Merriam-Webster Dictionary*, 1991). Habits can be positive – for example, brushing your teeth twice a day, taking a morning walk – or negative – for example, biting your nails or picking a scab. Negative habits are very common and can be difficult to extinguish. Although some negative habits may be considered to be a type of compulsion, presenting with a habit does not indicate a definitive diagnosis of an OCD-related disorder.

BEHAVIORS RELATED TO MEDICATIONS

It is important to be aware that some medications may have neuro-behavioral side effects. When new OCD-related behaviors or tics are observed, it is important to review a child's medication history to explore whether the behavior may be a side effect of the medication.

CASE STUDIES

Sophia admitted to her parents that she had been pulling out the hair on her head and also her eyebrow hairs. She reported that she was embarrassed of this behavior but unable to stop. In response to being asked why she pulled her hair, she reported that she felt a "tension in her body" which appeared to be briefly relieved when she pulled out her hair. Sophia's pediatrician obtained a thorough history and completed a full physical exam. Sophia was diagnosed with trichotillomania, which is considered an OCD-related disorder. She was referred to a psychologist.

Jack's parents met with a psychologist. The psychologist agreed that Jack was demonstrating a compulsive behavior. However, the psychologist also reported that compulsive behaviors are frequently observed in children with ASD. It was felt that Jack's new compulsive behavior was one more "piece of Jack's ASD puzzle," and it was not felt that this behavior required an additional diagnosis of OCD.

The developmental pediatrician who was following **Levi** obtained a thorough history and completed a full physical and neurological exam. It was noted that although Levi had presented with a motor tic prior to being treated with a stimulant medication, his skin picking was observed only after he began treatment. It was decided that his psychostimulant medication would be held and Levi would be monitored closely.

TREATMENT OF OCD AND OCD-RELATED DISORDERS

Behavioral Therapy

Behavioral therapy for childhood-onset OCD and OCD-related disorders typically includes cognitive behavioral therapy (CBT) and exposure response prevention (ERP). ERP is a therapy that includes exposing a person to the situations that provoke their obsessions and the associated distress while helping them prevent their compulsive responses, with the goal of breaking them from their obsessive-compulsive cycle (Koran et al., 2007). Multiple meta-analyses have found a combination of CBT and ERP to be effective in reducing OCD symptoms, with efficacy at least as effective in children and adolescents as in adults, and improvement in symptoms maintained after treatment (Farrell et al., 2023).

Medication

Although behavioral therapy is the first line of treatment for childhood OCD, treatment with medication has also been shown to be effective, with some selective serotonin reuptake inhibitor (SSRI) medications approved for children younger than ten years old (Nagata et al., 2022).

Combination Behavioral Therapy and Medication

Studies have found that treatment of moderate to severe childhood-onset OCD responds best to a combination of medication (selective serotonin reuptake inhibitors [SSRIs]) and behavioral therapy (Garcia et al., 2010). The randomized controlled Pediatric OCD Treatment Study (POTS) in 2004 evaluated the efficacy of CBT, the SSRI sertraline, and the combination of CBT and sertraline vs. placebo for children and adolescents with OCD, aged 7–17 years old. Improvements were observed in all three groups compared to placebo, with the most significant improvements in the combination group (POTS Team, 2004). A follow-up study was completed in 2011, the Pediatric OCD Treatment Study II (POTS II), which assessed treatment with SSRI only, SSRI and CBT "instruction" (CBT instructions given by a psychiatrist), and medication management with CBT (multiple sessions given by a therapist/psychologist). Medication management with CBT showed a significantly greater proportion of participants who responded to treatment (68.6% for medications and CBT, 34.0% for medications and instruction in CBT, and 30.0% for medication alone) (Franklin et al., 2011).

Results of a recent meta-analysis of treatments for OCD in children and adolescents revealed that exposure and response prevention therapy (both in-person and virtual), SSRI medications, and clomipramine are all effective in treating OCD. Moreover, exposure and response prevention therapy, either alone or in combination with treatment with an SSRI, appeared to be more effective than treatment with an SSRI alone (Steele et al., 2025).

TREATMENT OF TICS

Children who present with simple tics typically only require monitoring, guidance, and parental education. Calling attention to a child's tics should be discouraged. In some children, tics may be precipitated by stress, and calling attention to the tics can sometimes make a child self-conscious or anxious. Parents and teachers should be informed that tics are relatively common, and that the child is not demonstrating these movements or vocalizations to receive attention or to intentionally bother others. It should be noted that although tics are considered involuntary, sometimes individuals can prevent a tic with great effort. There are also therapists trained in comprehensive behavioral intervention for tics (CBIT), also known as "habit reversal therapy" (Bennett et al., 2020).

Overall, children who present with simple tics usually do not require specific therapies or medication. However, some children may present with more severe tics, including some with chronic tic disorders or Tourette syndrome, that interfere with their functioning – for example, their tics are so frequent and severe that they are unable to sit and complete their school work. These children will likely require further evaluation with exploration of treatments. Medical management of tics can be challenging. Medication trials may include alpha agonists, guanfacine or clonidine, and sometimes other psychiatric medications.

AUTHORS' COMMENTARY

Tics are not uncommon in children, including children with ADHD. Although there has been some concern that treatment with psychostimulant medication may precipitate tics, data suggest that there has not been consistently strong, definitive evidence to support a direct association between new onset or worsening of tics and stimulant treatment (Cohen et al., 2015).

However, if a child's tics appear to worsen at the same time as treatment with psychostimulant medication, it is typically considered appropriate that an alternative medication be considered.

Negative habits can be challenging to break. We have found that strategies are often more likely to be successful if the child has input into which specific strategy is going to be tried. For example, if the treatment plan includes a substitute strategy to decrease nail biting, "brain storming" with the child what might be a good substitute behavior (for example, pulling on an elastic wrist band) may increase the likelihood of success.

CASE STUDIES

Sophia was referred to a therapist who worked with her using cognitive-behavioral strategies. The therapy was helpful for a period of time, but Sophia's hair pulling returned. Sophia was referred to a child psychiatrist, and she continued to work with a psychologist who was trained in CBT and ERP. Sophia's psychiatrist began treatment with an SSRI medication. Sophia's trichotillomania decreased over time. However, Sophia periodically developed some other compulsive behaviors and continued to work with the psychologist and psychiatrist throughout middle and high school.

Jack received in-school and in-home applied behavior analysis (ABA) therapy, and addressing his compulsion with paper was included as a goal. In addition, Jack's father asked Jack for "assistance" in a building project. A box with slots was created, and Jack was asked to attempt to substitute placing paper into radiator gratings with placing paper into the box.

After **Levi's** stimulant medication was discontinued, his skin picking gradually decreased and eventually resolved. Levi's features of ADHD were reported to be negatively impacting on his functioning at school, so he was started on a trial of a nonstimulant medication, which was helpful. Levi continued to be treated with a nonstimulant ADHD medication throughout his schooling. His eye-blinking gradually decreased and resolved by middle school. His skin picking did not recur.

HANDOUT FOR CAREGIVERS

Obsessive Compulsive Disorder (OCD) and OCD-Related Disorders

Repetitive thoughts and actions can be part of normal childhood development. However, if your child's repetitive thoughts and actions appear excessive, are negatively impacting on their daily functioning, and cause stress, this may be cause for concern. If you are worried about your child's repetitive thoughts and behaviors, the first step is to discuss your concerns with your child's primary care provider, who may refer your child for further evaluation by a mental health professional.

Treatment

The first line of treatment for OCD is typically cognitive behavioral therapy (CBT). Children are taught to understand their fears and behaviors and learn techniques to gain control over their obsessive thoughts and behaviors. Exposure response prevention therapy is a form of CBT that involves very gradually exposing an individual to their obsessions while resisting the associated compulsive, ritualistic behaviors. Medication may also be prescribed. Family members and other people involved in your child's life will be important components of your child's treatment plan.

Tics

Tics are short, recurrent, involuntary movements (motor tics) or vocalizations (vocal tics). Tics are very common in school-aged children and may include eye blinking, shoulder shrugging, sniffling, coughing, or throat clearing.

Children who present with simple tics typically only require monitoring, guidance, and adult/family education. People involved in your child's life should be discouraged from calling attention to a child's tics. In some children, tics may be precipitated by stress, and calling attention to the tics can sometimes make a child anxious. Relatives and teachers should be informed that tics are relatively common and that the child is not demonstrating these movements or vocalizations to receive attention or to intentionally bother others.

Habits

Negative habits can be challenging to break. Strategies are often more likely to be successful if the child has input into which specific strategy is going to be tried. For example, if the treatment plan includes a substitute strategy to decrease nail biting, "brain storming" with the child what might be a good substitute behavior (for example, pulling on an elastic wrist band) can increase the likelihood of success.

It is important to note that some medications may have behavioral side effects. When a new behavior is observed, such as tics or OCD characteristics, it is important for you to discuss your child's medications with their primary care physician to explore whether the behaviors may be a side effect of the medication.

BIBLIOGRAPHY

Adam, G. P., Caputo, E. L., Kanaan, G., Freeman, J. B., Brannan, E. H., Balk, E. M., Trikalinos, T. A., & Steele, D. W. (2025). Brief assessment tools for obsessive-compulsive disorders in children: A systematic review. *Pediatrics*, 155(3): e2024068993. doi: 10.1542/peds.2024-068993.

American Psychiatric Association (APA) (2013). *Diagnostic and Statistical Manual of Mental Disorders – 5th edition*. Arlington, VA.: American Psychiatric Association Publishing.

Anxiety and Depression Association of America: Obsessive Compulsive Foundation Support Group: OCD at School. www.adaa.org.

Bennett, S. M., Capriotti, M., Bauer, C., Chang, S., Keller, A. E., Walkup, J., Woods, D., & Piacentini, J. (2020). Development and open trial of a psychosocial intervention for young children with chronic tics: The CBIT-JR study. *Journal of Behavioral Therapy and Experimental Psychiatry*, 51(4): 659–669. https://doi.org/10.1016/j.beth.2019.10.004. Epub 2019 Nov 27.

Cohen, S., Mulqueen, J., Ferracioli-Oda, E., Stuckelman, Z., Coughlin, C., Leckman, J., & Bloch M. (2015). Meta analysis: Risk of tics associated with stimulant use in randomized, placebo-controlled trials. *Journal of the American Academy of Child & Adolescent Psychiatry*, 54(9): 728–736. https://doi.org/10.1016/j.jaac.2015.06.011. Epub 2015 Jul 2.

Farrell, L. J., Waters, A. M., Storch, E. A., Simcock, G., Perkes, I. E., Grisham, J. R., Dyason, K. M., & Ollendick, T. H. (2023). Closing the gap for children with OCD: A staged-care model of cognitive behavioural therapy with exposure and response prevention. *Clinical Child and Family Psychology Review*, 26(3): 642–664. https://doi.org/10.1007/s10567-023-00439-2.

Franklin, M., Sapyta, J., Freeman, J. B., Khanna, M., Compton, S., Almirall, D., Moore, P., Choate-Summers, M., Garcia, A., Edson, A. L., Foa, E. B., March, J. S. (2011). Cognitive behavior therapy augmentation of pharmacotherapy in pediatric obsessive-compulsive disorder: The Pediatric OCD Treatment Study II (POTS II) randomized controlled trial. *Journal of the American Medical Association*, 306(11): 1224–1232. https://doi.org/10.1001/jama.2011.1344.

Garcia A. M., Sapyta J. J., Moore P. S., Freeman J. B., Franklin M. E., March J. S., Foa, E. B. (2010). Predictors and moderators of treatment outcome in pediatric obsessive compulsive treatment study (POTS I). *Journal of the American Academy of Child & Adolescent Psychiatry*, 49(10): 1024–1033. https://doi.org/10.1016/j.jaac.2010.06.013. Epub 2010 Sep 6.

Geller, D. A., Homayoun, S., & Johnson, G. (2021). Developmental considerations in obsessive compulsive disorder: Comparing pediatric and adult-onset cases. *Frontiers in Psychiatry*, 12: 678538. https://doi.org/10.3389/fpsyt.2021.678538.

International OCD Foundation. https://iocdf.org.

Koran L. M., Hanna G. L., Hollander, E., Nestadt, G., Simpson, H. B. (2007) Practice guidelines for treatment of patients with obsessive-compulsive disorder. *American Psychiatric Association*, http://www.psych.org/psych_pract/treatg/pg/prac_guide.cfm.

Merriam-Webster Dictionary (1991). Springfield, MA: Merriam-Webster Inc.

Morrison, J. (2014). *DSM-5 Made Easy. The Clinician's Guide to Diagnosis.* New York, NY: The Guilford Press.

Nagata, J. M., Chu J., Zamora, G., Ganson, K., Testa, A., Jackeson, D. B., Costello, C., Murray S. B., & Baker, F. C. (2022). Screen time and obsessive-compulsive disorder among children 9–10 years old: A prospective cohort study. *Journal of Adolescent Health*, 72: 390–396.

Nazeer, A., Latif, F., Mondal, A. Azeem, M. W., & Greydanus, D. E. (2020). Obsessive-compulsive disorder in children and adolescents: Epidemiology, diagnosis and management. *Translational Pediatrics*, 9(Suppl 1): S76–S93. doi: 10.21037/tp.2019.10.02.

Nelson, E. C., Hanna, G. L., Hudziak, J. J., Botteron, K. N., Heath, A. C., & Todd, R. D. (2001). Obsessive-compulsive scale of the child behavior checklist: Specificity, sensitivity, and predictive power. *Pediatrics*, 108(1): E14. https://doi.org/10.1542/peds.108.1.e14.

Obsessive-Compulsive Foundation, Inc. www.ocfoundation.org.

Pediatric OCD Treatment Study (POTS) Team (2004). Cognitive-behavior therapy, sertraline, and their combination for children and adolescents with obsessive-compulsive disorder: The pediatric OCD treatment study (POTS) randomized controlled trial. *Journal of the American Medical Association*, 292(16): 1969–1976. https://doi.org/10.1001/jama.292.16.1969.

Scahill, L., Riddle, M. A., McSwiggin-Hardin, M., Ort, S. I., King, R. A., Goodman, W. K., Cicchetti, D., & Leckman, J. F. (1997). Children's Yale-Brown obsessive compulsive scale: Reliability and validity. *Journal of the American Academy of Child & Adolescent Psychiatry*, 36(6): 844–852. https://doi.org/10.1097/00004583-199706000-00023.

Steele, D. W., Kanaan, G., Caputo, E. L., Freeman, J. B., Brannan, E. H., Balk, E. M., Trikalinos, T. A., & Adam, G. P. (2025). Treatment of obsessive-compulsive disorder in children and youth: A meta-analysis. *Pediatrics*, 155(3): e2024068992. https://doi.org/10.1542/peds.2024-068992.

Stewart, S. E., Rosario, M. C., Baer, L., Jenike, M. A., Geller, D. A., & Pauls, D. L. (2008). Four-factor structure of obsessive-compulsive disorder symptoms in children, adolescents, and adults. *Journal of the American Academy of Child & Adolescent Psychiatry*, 47(7): 763–772. https://doi.org/10.1097/CHI.0b013e318172ef1e.

Tourette Association of America. https://tourette.org.

Zohar A. H. (1999). The epidemiology of obsessive-compulsive disorder in children and adolescents. *Child and Adolescent Psychiatric Clinics*, 8(3): 445–460.

CHAPTER 11

Posttraumatic Stress Disorder or Just Some Challenging Experiences?

It has likely become clear from the previous chapters that many behaviors can be shared by multiple developmental-behavioral diagnoses, and sometimes can be considered within the scope of typical childhood behaviors. This can make arriving at a definitive diagnosis challenging. Symptoms such as inattention, distractibility, poor organizational skills, social skill difficulties, decreased eye contact, restricted range of affect, suboptimal school performance, irritability, sadness, anxiety, a decreased interest in activities, a regression in skills, and sleep disturbances, are symptoms that can result in caregiver and/or teacher concerns; and these are symptoms of multiple diagnoses. So, just to add to the diagnostic challenge, this chapter will discuss how all of these concerns can also be symptoms of trauma- and stressor-related disorders, including the diagnosis of posttraumatic stress disorder (PTSD).

Previous chapters have also indicated that a complex social and family history places a child at an increased risk for multiple developmental-behavioral diagnoses. Children can be very resilient, and some children appear to recover from negative and even traumatic experiences without meeting criteria for a specific mental health or behavioral diagnosis. However, sometimes traumatic experience(s) can be associated with one or more mental health issues, including the diagnosis of PTSD.

Let us discuss three children who are "not acting right."

CASE STUDIES

Grace is nine years old. She has always appeared cautious. She is a good student, but her fourth grade teacher has observed that recently Grace has

DOI: 10.4324/9781003639121-11

not been as social with the other students at school. During recess Grace has been sitting alone and not engaging with her friends despite their invitations to join them. She has not been volunteering in class, and she has not been completing her assignments. These are new concerns.

John is seven years old and attending second grade. His family recently relocated to the school district, so John is a new student in his class. He has been observed to be very reserved, with limited eye contact. This was initially felt to be likely related to him being a new student, as most of the other students in his class attended kindergarten and first grade together at the same school. However, John's affect has appeared flat; he has been observed to be unfocused, and he has not been completing his assignments. On a few occasions, John appeared to be staring off and "in his own world." The school nurse mentioned that this can sometimes be a presentation of absence seizures. John's mother was contacted and agreed to discuss this with John's new pediatrician.

Mason is four years old. He was adopted from an orphanage in eastern Europe six months ago. His parents were advised to enroll him in a preschool that included an English Language Learner program. Mason has been observed to be overly active at school and at home; his ability to focus is limited. He has started learning English, and, with redirection and support, he has gradually been able to sit and participate in some group activities at school. Mason's preschool teacher has expressed a concern that Mason may be presenting with features of ADHD, but she also feels that it is possible that his high activity level may be related to his past experiences in an orphanage.

PTSD

PTSD is diagnosis related to a negative psychological reaction to a traumatic experience. Examples of potentially traumatic events can include an accident or injury, violent acts, neglect or abandonment, death of a loved one, environmental disasters, and acts of abuse. Symptoms may include re-experiencing the trauma (for example, through memories of the event or feeling as if the event is happening again); attempting to avoid external reminders of the trauma; negative emotions, such as agitation and detachment from others; social withdrawal; and other symptoms, such as irritability, anger, self-destructive behavior, hypervigilance, poor concentration, and sleep disturbances (Ringeisen et al., 2016).

A child's age and developmental level, temperament, and previous history of trauma can influence the range of difficulties a child may experience following a traumatic event. Additionally, other risk and possible protective factors (for example, the kind of support the child has at home and from other adults) can impact the child's ability to respond and cope with the challenges they may experience following a traumatic event (Morrison, 2014; Ringeisen et al., 2016; Scheerings, 2011). A qualified professional must conduct a thorough assessment of the child's behavior to provide a diagnosis of PTSD.

The impact of early trauma can sometimes affect a child's daily life long after the traumatic event has ended. Symptoms can vary according to developmental stage. A toddler or preschooler may lose previously acquired skills, such as toileting or language skills, and an older child/adolescent may demonstrate unusually aggressive or self-destructive behavior. Evidence of their negative memories can sometimes be verbalized by school-age children and adolescents, but may be disclosed by preschoolers through play. Some symptoms/behaviors may include avoidance behaviors, restricted range of affect, diminished interest in activities, detachment from loved ones, difficulty concentrating, and irritability/outbursts of anger – there may also be differences in presentation depending on the child's age and developmental level. An evaluator therefore needs an understanding of child development in order to use appropriate methods to explore the child's symptoms. Obtaining a detailed history requires expertise, time, and effort.

According to the National Center for PTSD, about 15% to 43% of girls and 1% to 6% of boys experience at least one traumatic event. Of those children and adolescents who have experienced trauma, 3% to 15% of girls and 1% to 6% of boys develop PTSD, with differences noted depending on the type of trauma experienced (National Center for PTSD, n.d. – a).

CASE STUDIES

Grace's teacher met with Grace and inquired about her home life. Grace disclosed that the family was forced to leave their rented apartment as they were no longer able to afford to pay the rent. The family had been living with various friends and family members from week to week for the past two months. Grace reported that she was worried about her parents and her two siblings, especially her youngest brother who was only a year old. Grace's parents were contacted and agreed to meet with the staff at school.

The school social worker notified a community group that was able to assist the family in finding public housing and other supports. Grace's affect began to improve.

John received an electroencephalogram (EEG), which revealed no evidence of seizures. During recess, two students got into a physical altercation; the altercation was broken up, but John was found hiding behind a tree shaking. With John's mother's permission, the school adjustment counselor began meeting with John twice a week. John's mother also confided with the staff at school that she and John had "gone through a lot" prior to moving to their new home.

Initially John was not very interactive, but he began to relax and feel more comfortable and enjoyed playing board games with the school counselor. John disclosed that he was very worried about his mother. The counselor initially suspected that John may be exhibiting features of an anxiety disorder. She felt strongly that more intensive counseling outside of school was needed. John's mother reported that she was working with her own counselor but would also schedule John for individual counseling outside of school. She also confided to the school counselor that she was previously the victim of domestic violence to which John had been a witness.

Mason worked with a counselor, and play therapy was incorporated into his sessions. Mason's home life was positive. Although information about his experience at the orphanage was fairly limited, his parents had spent two weeks there before bringing Mason home, and had been fairly comfortable with the environment. The orphanage was understaffed but the staff appeared to genuinely care about the children.

The teacher had a volunteer sit next to Mason during classroom activities to provide redirection and support. It was observed at school and at home that Mason's eye contact and his ability to focus and pay attention gradually improved. He enjoyed attention from adults and he began engaging in play with other children. By the end of the school year, there were less concerns regarding the diagnosis of ADHD.

FEATURES OF PTSD THAT OVERLAP WITH OTHER DIAGNOSES

As stated previously, just about all the diagnoses covered in the previous chapters can share some symptoms with PTSD. These overlapping symptoms can make it difficult to obtain a correct diagnosis, which can complicate both assessment and treatment. This is especially true if a child's family and social histories have not been completely revealed. The complexity of the child's symptoms and presentation can sometimes lead to multiple diagnoses and potential misdiagnoses, particularly when the impact of the child's trauma history goes unrecognized. Some children may therefore receive treatment with unnecessary medications and/or therapies. Examples of some diagnoses whose symptoms overlap with symptoms of PTSD include the following.

- **Attention-deficit/hyperactivity disorder (ADHD)**: Difficulty concentrating and learning in school, distractibility, poor listening skills, disorganization, hyperactivity, and restlessness.
- **Anxiety**: Restlessness, agitation, social challenges, poor concentration, poor sleep.
- **Depression**: Sadness, withdrawal, anger, poor concentration, and a decreased interest in things that were previously enjoyable.
- **Learning disability**: Poor school performance and difficulty focusing.

It is essential that an evaluator spend a great deal of time with a child and obtain a thorough history – sorting out a definitive diagnosis takes expertise and time.

Let us add one more complication to the complexity of childhood trauma. It is possible for a child to have more than one diagnosis, as the diagnosis of PTSD increases a child's risk of meeting criteria for other mental health diagnosis, including ADHD, anxiety, learning challenges, and depression. The existence of co-morbid diagnoses can add challenges to assessment and treatment. It has been reported that children with co-morbid diagnoses of ADHD and PTSD have an increased risk of additional psychiatric disorders, leading to more severe outcomes. It has also been reported that symptoms of PTSD may exacerbate symptoms of other mental health diagnoses, which has the potential to worsen a child's functioning at home, at school, and among peers. However, on a more positive note, treating a child's other mental health diagnosis, such as ADHD, may result in an improvement in the child's treatment for trauma and their outcome (Ringeisen et al., 2016; Siegfried & Blackshear, 2016).

ASSESSMENT FOR PTSD

Since symptoms of PTSD overlap with multiple other diagnoses, professionals should make sure they consider the possibility of childhood trauma in children they are evaluating for other diagnoses. Self-report of a history of trauma is unlikely to be provided spontaneously by a child. A thorough, systematic, and age-appropriate exploration of a child's history is therefore needed, and this requires time and the establishment of a positive, comfortable rapport with the child. If childhood trauma is suspected, a specific assessment by a professional with expertise in this area should be requested.

A comprehensive assessment for childhood trauma includes a thorough exploration of events in the child's past that may have been traumatic, including at what developmental stage the events took place; symptoms that have been exhibited by the child and apparent precipitants of the symptoms; and the child's family and social history. Information should be obtained from multiple sources using a variety of techniques – for example, interviews with the child, caregivers, sometimes relatives, teachers and therapists. Behavioral observations of the child during their evaluation, including their play, and use of standardized assessment tools are important components of the assessment and should be repeated over time as the child becomes more comfortable with the evaluator. It is also important to explore the child's strengths and system of emotional support in order to assist in assessing their potential capacity for resilience (Siegfried & Blackshear, 2016).

OTHER STRESSOR-RELATED DISORDERS

Acute Stress Disorder

Symptoms of an acute distress disorder can be similar to PTSD but occur right after the traumatic event and do not last as long (American Psychiatric Association (APA), 2013; Morrison, 2014).

Reactive Attachment Disorder (RAD)

Reactive attachment disorder can be a result of negative child care experiences – this can include physical or emotional abuse or neglect. The child is observed to withdraw emotionally and neither seeks out nor responds to comfort and affection from an adult. The child can appear sad or sometimes irritable. Externalizing types of symptoms can also be observed (APA, 2013; Morrison, 2014).

Disinhibited Social Engagement Disorder

This mental health diagnosis can also result from an experience of abuse or neglect by a child's caregivers. These children demonstrate an unusually strong comfort level with unfamiliar adults (APA, 2013; Morrison, 2014).

Adjustment Disorder

A child with an adjustment disorder presents with behavioral symptoms, and sometimes symptoms of depression and/or anxiety, in response to a stressor. Their symptoms are considered more severe than would be expected of most children at their age and developmental level (APA, 2013; Morrison, 2014).

Prolonged Grief Disorder

Prolonged grief disorder (introduced in Chapter 9) was a diagnosis added to the 2022 revised *Diagnostic and Statistical Manual of Mental Disorders – 5th edition* (DSM-5-TR5). Grief is a natural response after the death of a loved one. Prolonged grief disorder is diagnosed when the response to the death of a loved one is more intense, severe, and prolonged than would be considered typical for the child's age (APA, 2022).

TREATMENT OF PTSD

Treatment of PTSD should be provided by professionals who have expertise in this diagnosis. A child's specific treatment depends on different factors, such as the child's age, developmental level, the specific trauma, and the timing and degree of their exposure to the traumatic event(s). Many children may not initially feel comfortable discussing their trauma history, and the evaluator must be prepared to advance at a very gradual pace that is comfortable for the child. Some of the components of trauma treatment include teaching stress management and relaxation techniques, particularly to deal with reminders/triggers of their experience; encouraging routines to make the child feel safe and secure; helping a child learn to gain more control over regulating their emotions, behavior, and physiological response to stressors; and enabling a child to gradually talk about their traumatic events to assist them in learning to cope with the memories and gain control of their pain and stress (Siegfried & Blackshear, 2016). Some specific types of therapies include the following.

Trauma-Focused Cognitive Behavioral Therapy (CBT)

This type of therapy can be provided for children from the age of three through adolescence, who present with a history of trauma. In addition to CBT techniques, such as relaxation and self-understanding of triggers and behavior, the therapy includes education about trauma, parenting skills that can help the child, and methods to help the child to understand the connections between their feelings and behaviors and the traumatic event. Research studies have reported benefits of this type of therapy (Vanderzee et al., 2018).

Parent-Child Interaction Therapy

This therapy addresses behavioral problems exhibited by relatively young children, typically aged two to seven. It can be implemented to address some behavioral issues presented by children who have experienced trauma (Vanderzee et al., 2018).

Child Parent Psychotherapy

This is a relationship-based therapy for infants and young children who have experienced trauma. Issues, such as attachment, can be addressed as part of this therapy (Vanderzee et al., 2018).

Trauma Systems Therapy

This is a therapy model for children that addresses the child's individual needs in the context of their social environment. The model utilizes a multi-disciplinary approach to care (The National Child Traumatic Stress Network, n.d.).

Pharmacotherapy

Medications are sometimes recommended for children who have experienced trauma, typically to treat symptoms of other diagnoses that may exist alongside PTSD – for example, ADHD, depression, and anxiety (Siegfried & Blackshear, 2016).

CASE STUDIES

Grace's family was provided with multiple community resources. Both of her parents eventually found employment. Grace and her sibling participated in an after-school program, and Grace's grandparents watched Grace's infant brother while her parents were at work. Grace's affect improved. Grace was a strong student and received a scholarship to attend college after she graduated high school.

John began working with a counselor who specialized in childhood trauma. He was diagnosed with PTSD and his story was gradually uncovered: John had watched his mother being physically abused by his biological father since for as long as he could remember. After each incident he would try to help his mother, giving her hugs and kisses. The police had been contacted multiple times, but his mother did not press charges and made excuses for the father's behavior (possibly out of fear). The abuse finally reached a point that resulted in John and his mother residing temporarily in a Women's Shelter. John's father was arrested and imprisoned after becoming involved in a bar fight that resulted in a death. John was aware that his father was incarcerated. John and his mother moved to a new apartment in a new city.

John worked intensively with the counselor. He continued to express fear for his mother. However, his behavior and social skills gradually showed some improvement. Although his features of PTSD gradually decreased, John continued to meet with a counselor throughout elementary, middle, and high school.

Although **Mason's** organizational skills and attention continued to be relative weaknesses during elementary school, it was not felt that he met criteria for ADHD or PTSD. A core evaluation revealed some executive functioning weaknesses, and a 504 Accommodation Plan was created. During the latter part of elementary school, Mason's 504 Accommodation Plan was able to be discontinued. Mason successfully attended a vocational high school.

Final note: All children have natural resilience and strengths. These strengths, in combination with supports from caring adults and professionals, can provide tools to assist them in learning to adapt to life stressors.

HANDOUT FOR CAREGIVERS

Posttraumatic Stress Disorder (PTSD)

PTSD is a mental health diagnosis that is the result of physical and/or emotional trauma. The disorder can last for an extended period of time after the trauma has occurred. Children can show a variety of symptoms. Younger children are often unable to verbalize their thoughts and feelings and can present with disruptive behavior or significant separation anxiety.

Treatment

Working with a counselor/therapist who has specialized expertise in working with children with a history of trauma is vitally important, and family supports should also be accessed. A multidisciplinary team of professionals working with your child and family is beneficial.

How to Help Your Child

Parents/caregivers will typically try to do everything to prevent their child from experiencing trauma, but some events will be out of your control. However, there are strategies that families can use to provide children with some "life skill" tools – for example, it is important for children to learn that they should say "no" to people who try to touch them in a way that makes them feel uncomfortable, and that they should inform a parent, relative, teacher, or other trusted adult if this happens.

BIBLIOGRAPHY

American Psychiatric Association (APA) (2013). *Diagnostic and Statistical Manual of Mental Disorders – 5th edition*. Arlington, VA: American Psychiatric Association Publishing.

American Psychiatry Association (APA) (2022). *Diagnostic and Statistical Manual of Mental Disorders – 5th edition. Text Revision (DSM-5-TR)*. American Psychiatric Association Publishing.

Morrison, J. (2014). *DSM-5 Made Easy. The Clinician's Guide to Diagnosis*. New York, NY: The Guilford Press.

National Center for PTSD (n.d. – a). *How common is PTSD in children and teens?* www.ptsd.va.gov.

National Center for PTSD (n.d. – b). *PTSD in children and teens*. www.ptsd.va.gov.

The National Child Traumatic Stress Network (n.d.). (https://www.nctsn.org).

Ringeisen, H., Casanueva, C., Stambaugh, L., Bose, J., Hedden, S. (2016). *DSM-5 changes: Implications for child serious emotional disturbance* [Unpublished internal documentation]. Rockville, Maryland: Center for Behavioral Health Statistics and Quality. Substance Abuse and Mental Health Service Administration (US).

Scheerings, M. S. (2011). PTSD in children younger than the age of 13: Toward developmentally sensitive assessment and management. *Journal of Child & Adolescent Trauma*, 41(3): 181–197. https://doi.org/10.1080/19361521.2011.597079.

Siegfried, C. B., & Blackshear, K. (2016). *Is it ADHD or child traumatic stress? A guide for clinicians*. Los Angeles, CA & Durham, NC: National Child Traumatic Stress Network, with assistance from the National Resource Center on ADHD: A program of children and adults with attention-deficit/hyperactivity disorder (CHADD).

Vanderzee, K. L., Sigel, B. A., Pemberton, J. R., & John, S. G. (2018). Treatments for early childhood trauma: Decision considerations for clinicians. *Journal of Child and Adolescent Trauma*, 12(4): 515–528. https://doi.org/10.1007/s40653-018-0244-6.

The National Child Traumatic Stress Network. www.nctsn.org.

CHAPTER 12

An Exploration of Parenting

Parenting is complex. It can be the most fulfilling yet difficult experience, and each parenting experience comes with its own set of unique challenges and rewards. Variations in parenting are based on numerous factors such as parent styles and practices, developmental stages, the temperament of the child, and the environmental and psychosocial stressors impacting the family unit. The parent–child relationship is always evolving. Understanding the factors that contribute to this complex relationship will enable you to help parents and caregivers achieve the best possible outcome for their child.

PARENTING STYLES

Parenting styles are defined as the emotional environments in which parents/caregivers raise their children. Parenting practices are specific actions caregivers employ in parenting. Diana Baumrind, a developmental psychologist, identified three initial parenting styles: authoritarian, permissive, and authoritative (1966). In the 1980s, Stanford researchers Eleanor Maccoby and John Martin added a fourth style, neglectful/uninvolved, to Baumrind's typology (1983). These four styles are often called the *Baumrind parenting styles* or *Maccoby and Martin parenting styles*. Parents often use a combination of these four parenting styles when raising their children (Vande Kemp, 2000; Maccoby & Martin, 1983).

Neglectful caregivers are unable to meet their child's emotional and physical needs appropriately. Caregivers who neglect their children require support to explore their own personal issues to determine if, with supports and assistance, they will be able to parent successfully.

DOI: 10.4324/9781003639121-12

Authoritarian parenting is characterized by the caregiver setting rigid rules and demanding obedience. They exert control over the child through power and coercion, sometimes using withdrawal of approval to have their child conform. This type of caregiver is described as a stern disciplinarian and sometimes lacks an understanding of their child's needs; however, caregivers who are considered "strict" or even "controlling," can also love their child and want the best for them. Outside influences, such as daycare providers, school personnel, therapists, family, and friends can ensure that a caregiver's strictness is not excessive and controlling, while educating parents to create a healthier family environment.

Permissive parenting, also known as indulgent parenting, is characterized by a great deal of parental warmth and few rules or boundaries. Limited demands are typically placed on the children, and these parents are often reluctant to enforce rules and meaningful consequences for misbehavior. Caregivers may be viewed as a friend more than a parental figure. Caregivers can be taught that setting limits can ultimately enhance their relationship with their child.

Authoritative caregivers set clear expectations for their child. They monitor their child's behavior, use discipline based on reasoning, and encourage their child to make decisions and learn from their mistakes. They are warm and nurturing, and they treat their child with kindness, respect, and affection.

Although the authoritative parenting style sets the standard for parenting, caregivers often employ the whole spectrum of styles, depending on the circumstances. For example, a caregiver can be more or less understanding at different times. Caregivers modify their style and practice based on the developmental stage and behavior of the child, the distinctive family unit, and what the caregiver is able to offer.

"Gentle Parenting"

Gentle parenting was identifed by Sarah Ockwell-Smith (2016). A more recent parenting style that arrived during the age of social media, it includes respect, empathy, and positive discipline.

CASE STUDIES

Jennifer reported that her parents had been strict. They had rigid rules and expected obedience, i.e., authoritarian parenting. She rebelled during her high school years by cutting classes and sneaking out of the house. She says she knew her parents loved her, but vowed she would never raise her child in that way.

When **Victoria** was born, Jennifer showered her with love. She set few rules and made minimal demands during Victoria's toddler and preschool years; she was a friend to Victoria. When Victoria was five years old, Jennifer reported that Victoria became "fresh" and oppositional at home. She was concerned as Victoria was now attending kindergarten and she worried that Victoria's behavior was problematic. Jennifer met with Victoria's teacher who reported that Victoria could sometimes be "bossy" toward her peers but responded to the rules and structure of the classroom. The teacher suggested that Jennifer join a parenting group offered in the community. Jennifer began to gradually establish some rules in the home: no talking back; no physical acting out; and three chances to follow a request. Victoria received a sticker every two hours for following the rules. Gradually Victoria showed improvement in her behavior at home. Jennifer transitioned from a permissive parenting style to an authoritative style.

TYPES OF PARENTS

AUTHORS' COMMENTARY

It is our hope that acceptance and support for different types of caregivers and their families will continue to expand. Only a selection of "types" of parents are included in this section.

Teen Parents

Pregnant teens are more likely to participate in regular prenatal care if they have the support of a caregiver (Lee & Grubbs, 1995). If support is lacking, prenatal care may be sporadic or non-existent. Pregnant teens are more likely to suffer complications during pregnancy. Their babies are more likely to experience premature birth, low birth weight, or serious health problems (Diabelková et al., 2023; March of Dimes, n.d.). The American Academy of Child and Adolescent Psychiatry notes that a teen parent may be at risk of feeling anxious and depressed about the future and the unfamiliar role of parenting. The biological father of the baby may not be involved in parenting the child. If an adolescent mother drops out of school, she may lack the skills necessary to secure gainful employment to support herself and her child.

Although teen parenting presents many obstacles, adolescents can still be successful parents. Teen parents should be encouraged to stay in school. Many schools offer programs for pregnant and parenting teens. Community supports, such as childcare, child development/parenting classes, and transportation resources will aid the adolescent parent. Counseling to address their emotional health, interpersonal relationships, and decision-making are most beneficial. The support of the teen's family members or other adult role models can be invaluable. With supportive services in place, both formal and informal, a teen parent can better understand the developmental stages of their child, embrace their role as a parent and provide a nurturing environment for their child.

Grandparents Raising Grandchildren

Grandparents raising their grandchildren has become more common. According to the U.S. Census Bureau, in 2015 there were 2.6 million grandparents raising their grandchildren. This is a 6% increase from the 2008 census report. This is a result of the grandparents' adult child being unable to parent. Substance abuse, mental health, physical health, incarceration, and/or domestic violence issues may be contributing factors. If the change in the caregiver role is unplanned, grandparents have to transition from the role of grandparent to parent quickly and sometimes with little preparation. Grandparents may harbor feelings of resentment, guilt, or disappointment toward their adult child. Older grandparents may have age-related health conditions and/or limited financial resources. As a result, grandparents may be at an increased risk for mental health challenges and face social isolation. Younger grandparents may be continuing to raise their own children while remaining in the workforce.

If the grandchild is fleeing a chaotic environment to be given care by their grandparents, they may have suffered abuse and neglect from their biological parent. The grandchild may feel rejected, guilty, and angry. They may demonstrate challenging behaviors such as aggression and acting out. School performance may begin to decline. Perhaps the child is conflicted about their relationship with their parents and the parenting role of their grandparents. In order to successfully support the family, community support service providers such as a pediatrician, school personnel, therapists, and child welfare agencies must consider the developmental stages of the child, any developmental diagnosis (for example, learning disabilities, attention-deficit/hyperactivity disorder [ADHD], etc.) given to the child prior to placement, as well as the needs of the grandparents.

It is also notable that grandparents have a unique advantage in their parenting roles. They have raised children once before, and they can use these life experiences as guideposts to providing care. Although this relationship can be complex, with the right tools and attitude, a positive outcome is achievable. Child welfare agencies may be involved and can assist with legal matters through methods such as retaining legal custody of the child while the grandparents retain physical custody. Agencies can assist grandparents in maintaining boundaries between themselves and their adult children for the benefit of the children. Child welfare agencies are often able to provide compensation to ease the financial burden of raising grandchildren. These agencies also have access to community services such as daycare, after school programs, camperships, and counseling resources for the family unit.

Grandparents may also opt to obtain legal guardianship of their grandchild and pursue supportive services for themselves and their grandchild, independent of the child welfare system.

Grandparents can benefit from parenting education to better understand current information related to child development, behaviors, and effective discipline techniques. Support groups serve as a helpful resource as well. These can be a support as well as a social outlet. If the child is of school age, the school system can help grandparents become familiar with what supportive services may be available for the child and for themselves. Most schools have adjustment counseling services as well as academic assistance available.

Grandparents sometimes may neglect themselves due to the responsibilities of raising their grandchildren. Grandparents need to be encouraged to maintain their physical and mental health by following up with their health-care providers as scheduled. The social network established by grandparents prior to the arrival of the grandchildren is important and should be maintained, even if that requires some modification. This will help prevent grandparents from isolating themselves socially. By remaining socially engaged and allowing for some rest and relaxation time, grandparents can reduce burnout and depression.

Grandparents and grandchildren should be encouraged to participate in "grandfamily" therapy. A therapist identifies the strengths and challenges of both the grandchild and grandparent to offer valuable strategies to build on the positive and reduce the negative. Grandparents will be able to gain insight into their grandchildren's feelings and behaviors, and the grandchildren will be able to share their feelings with a professional in a safe and neutral environment. Some agencies offer homebased counseling services.

This can be helpful as it allows the therapist to view the "grandfamily" in their own environment and minimizes scheduling and transportation issues.

Ongoing assessment and evaluation of this relationship is needed as circumstances change. A parent may obtain custody of their child; a grandparent's health may change; and the developmental, behavioral, and educational needs of the child may evolve resulting in the need for re-evaluation of supportive services to ensure the best possible outcomes for all.

Foster Parents

Foster parents open their homes to the most vulnerable children. Often, foster children have experienced abuse and/or neglect. Newborns may have a history of neonatal abstinence syndrome, prematurity, and/or other medically complex issues; some children may have been in numerous foster placements; siblings may have been separated; contact with their biological family could be problematic; older children could be aging out of the foster care system. A child's developmental and behavioral issues could be a result of any number of circumstances. It is important for the foster parent to work collaboratively with the child welfare agency. An agency social worker will be able to provide the foster parent with some background information on the child and assist with supportive services to address adjustment concerns. Child welfare agencies have access to specific community supports that may be used only by child welfare agencies. Services such as early intervention programs, after-school programs, intensive treatment programs, and foster parent support groups can be extremely valuable to both the foster child and the foster parent. Foster parents should be encouraged to take advantage of the services offered by the child welfare agency. This complex family system can be successful when a foster parent's parenting style is best characterized as authoritative; the foster child's developmental and behavioral needs are identified and being met; and supportive services are in place.

Single Parents

Single parents, whether by choice or as a result of divorce or death, have unique strengths and challenges. The responsibilities of sustaining financial security, providing a stable living environment, and caring for the physical and emotional needs of the child can be challenging. A child's development and behavior can be affected by parent stressors.

A single divorced parent may have the added strain of parental conflict, visitation problems, unrealistic expectations of the family functioning (attempting to continue to function as a two-parent family), and sometimes the introduction of a new person into the child's life. A parent may observe a change in the child's school performance, peer relationships, and behavior. It is not uncommon for children of divorce to act out or withdraw. Recognizing one's parenting style and practice and having insight into the child's stage of development and behavior is vital. This awareness will assist the single parent in identifying normal vs. abnormal adjustment and coping strengths and weaknesses of both the parent and the child. Seeking services from a mental health professional is a helpful option.

Single parents and their children benefit from the informal support network of family and friends. These informal support systems can be a social outlet for both parent and child, offering adult companionship and allowing the child to interact with other children. Also, there can be a sharing of resources among the group, such as babysitting, carpool options, and knowledge of community resources. This informal support system can act as an extended family to the parent and child.

Two-Parent Families

Two-parent families have the benefit of sharing the parental responsibilities of child-rearing. Although this is viewed as positive, two-parent families can also experience challenges. Parents may have the same parenting style, but different parenting practices. For example, parents may disagree on discipline techniques, one parent being the disciplinarian, the other being more lenient. Parents may view their child's development differently. One may not recognize developmental delays or be accepting of a professional diagnosis given to the child. When conflict erupts between parents, a child may respond to their parents' differences with challenging behavior. Having two different sets of rules and expectations within the home can be confusing and difficult for children.

Some couples are able to reflect on their parenting practices and the impact they have on their child and their partner. They are able to communicate their differences and make adjustments to benefit the family unit. At times, differences may be too difficult for parents to tackle on their own. If this is the case, the couple should consider professional intervention. Depending on the developmental stage of the child, family counseling can be helpful.

CREATING AND MAINTAINING A SUCCESSFUL TEAM

When parents and caregivers expect too much of themselves or their child, stress is almost always inevitable. You can best serve this population by being an active listener to gain an understanding of the family unit. It is important to ask: what is your family's definition of success? What is your family's definition of failure? How are success and failure measured, and by whom? What may be failure for one is success for another. The caregiver–child relationship should be considered a team. The complex relationship is an interdependent one. Caregivers must evaluate what success is for them.

The first step in creating a successful caregiver/child team is for the caregivers to understand their child's behavior and developmental stage. The child may be developing within normal limits. The child may exhibit challenging behaviors, but that does not mean those behaviors are abnormal, they might be normal variations. Alternatively, the child may display atypical behaviors that warrant professional assessment and/or intervention. The child may also have a diagnosed developmental disorder. Caregivers may ask, "How will I know the difference?" It has been our intent throughout this book to provide clinicians with the tools to help caregivers better understand a child's normal development, variations of normal development, and the characteristics suggestive of a specific developmental diagnosis.

The second step is for the caregiver to gain insight into their own parenting style and parenting practices as well as their own challenges and psycho-social stressors. It is important to recognize caregivers' style, strengths, and challenges to understand how these factors impact the relationship they have with their child.

The third step is to work together to achieve the best possible outcomes for the caregiver and their child. This can be achieved by recognizing the strengths and challenges of the team. Professionals should remind caregivers that seeking support, whether formal or informal, for all members of the team should be viewed as a strength, not a weakness. Professionals should be familiar with local resources and aware of the purpose, process, and procedures of applying for services. Seeking support will enable both child and caregiver to change and grow in a positive direction while strengthening their relationship.

The final step is to regularly monitor the success of the team and make adjustments as needed. Caregivers and children change over time, as do family dynamics and environmental situations. New stressors may come into play (family members die, children are born or adopted, divorce occurs, the family moves to a new town, etc.). As children mature and move into new developmental stages, they may benefit from changes in parenting practices. Once the child's needs are identified, appropriate actions can be taken to continue to support the caregiver/child team. Each caregiver/child relationship has its own unique strengths and challenges. There is no right or wrong, just what works for the specific caregiver–child team.

Final note: Parenting is complex. Having an understanding of the developmental and behavioral complexities of children, parenting styles, and unique family units enables the clinician to assist parents and children on their journey.

BIBLIOGRAPHY

American Academy of Child and Adolescent Psychiatry (n.d.). *Supporting pregnant parenting.* https://www.aacap.org.

American Association for Marriage and Family Therapy. Grandparents raising grandchildren. https://www.aamft.org/AAMFT/consumer_updates/grandparents.aspx.

Anderson, L. R., Hemez, P. F., & Kreider, R. M. (2022). Living arrangements of children: 2019. census.gov/content/dam/Census/library/publications/2022/demo/p70-174.pdf.

Baumrind, D. (1966). Effects of authoritative parental control on child behavior. *Child Development,* 37(4): 887–907. https://doi.org/10.2307/1126611.

Coontz, S. (1997). *The Way We Really Are: Coming to Terms With America's Changing Families.* New York: Basic Books.

Child Welfare Information Gateway. https://www.childwelfare.gov/topics/permanency/foster-care.

Diabelková, J., Rimárová, K., Dorko, E., Urdzík, P., Houžvičková, A., Argalášová, L. (2023). Adolescent pregnancy outcomes and risk factors. *International Journal of Environmental Research and Public Health,* 20(5): 4113. https://doi.org/10.3390/ijerph20054113.

Lee, S. H., & Grubbs, L. M. (1995). Pregnant teenagers' reasons for seeking or delaying prenatal care. *Clinical Nursing Research,* 4(1): 38–49. https://doi.org/10.1177/105477389500400105.

Maccoby, E., & Martin, J. (1983). Socialization in the context of the family: Parent-child interaction. In P. Mussen & E. M. Hetherington (Eds.), *Handbook of Child psychology, Volume IV: Socialization, Personality, and Social Development* (pp. 1–101). New York, NY: John Wiley.

March of Dimes (n.d.). Youth health education series: Teen2Teen. https://www.marchofdimes.org.

Ockwell-Smith, S. (2016). *The Gentle Parenting Book: How to Raise Calmer, Happier Children from Birth to Seven.* UK: Piatkus Books.

Positive Parenting Ally (n.d.). Twelve types of parenting styles and discipline strategies. www.positive-parenting-ally.com.

US Census Bureau. https://www.census.gov.

Urban, L., & Carreu, G. (2025) 8 common family structures in modern-day society https://www.wikihow.com/Types-of-Family.

Vande Kemp, H. (2000). Baumrind, Diana Blumberg. In L. Balter (Ed.), *Parenthood in America: An Encyclopedia* (pp. 80–84). Santa Barbara, Calif: ABC-CLIO.

CHAPTER 13

(More) Frequently Asked Questions

My child's speech is delayed...should I be worried?
It is clear from the information provided in the chapters in this book, that communication skill delays can be a presentation for multiple diagnoses, including autism spectrum disorder (ASD), an intellectual disability (ID), a hearing deficit, and a specific speech and/or language delay or disorder. As a general rule, a child who is delayed in their oral speech but is communicative, using nonverbal gestures, facial expressions, and sounds, is typically a more positive presentation than a child who makes no attempt to communicate. However, whenever there is a concern regarding a child's speech-language development, a referral for a hearing assessment and a speech-language evaluation is recommended.

My child's motor skills are delayed...should I be worried?
A delay in motor development can also be associated with multiple diagnoses. As described in Chapter 1, the way a child moves is important when exploring reasons for a child's motor delays. Is their muscle tone decreased? Are their muscles weak? Are they poorly coordinated? Have other first-degree relatives presented similarly and what was their later development? The first steps are typically for a child's primary care physician to complete a physical and neurological examination and also make a referral for an evaluation by an early intervention program. Based on the results, further evaluation may be indicated.

Is my child's behavior inappropriate or is it just that I have a low tolerance for what is considered typical childhood behavior?
There is no perfect parent – acknowledging your own challenges and how they may impact your child can often be helpful in understanding your child's behavior.

DOI: 10.4324/9781003639121-13

If the feedback you receive from other adults who interact with your child, particularly their teachers, is positive, then you can be reassured that your child is able to behave appropriately. However, children often demonstrate more challenging behavior with their parents vs. other adults, particularly in a safe home environment. If your child's behavior appears problematic at home and has created parental frustration and/or stress, then seeking professional guidance is typically beneficial in order to clarify:

- whether the behavior you have observed at home is significantly problematic and why this behavior is being demonstrated only at home;
- how to best respond to what is considered "typical" child misbehavior;
- whether your own stress level is negatively impacting on your ability to deal with your child's behavior.

Does my child need medication?

If you have not received negative feedback from your child's teacher regarding their behavior, it is unlikely that your child is in need of treatment with medication.

If your child's behavior, including a high activity level, impulsivity, and limited attention span, is not negatively impacting on their functioning, particularly during school, it is unlikely that your child is in need of treatment with medication.

Before a trial of treatment with medication is initiated, it is important to try to explore whether there is a specific reason for their behavior that can be addressed without medication.

- Is your child's difficulty paying attention in school a result of a learning disability, a communication disorder, or a processing disorder? It is difficult to pay attention to instructions/lessons that you do not understand.
- Is your child's behavior related to a traumatic event?
- Is your child's behavior a way for them seek attention (even if the attention is not positive)?

Why have the professionals not agreed on my child's diagnosis?

Although there are clinical criteria that are established for developmental and mental health diagnoses, professionals may not always completely agree on whether a child meets criteria for a specific diagnosis. This may be related to the following:

- definitions of/criteria for specific diagnoses may have changed over time;
- there are often no specific objective diagnostic tests (blood test, neuroimaging) for mental health diagnoses;
- children may present differently for different evaluators.

Why has a specific diagnosis not been identified?

Although there may be several reasons why a specific diagnosis may not have been identified, two relatively common reasons include are listed below.

- Although a child experiences differences/weaknesses/challenges, these may not appear to be significant enough to meet criteria for a specific diagnosis.
- If a child's differences/weaknesses/challenges do not negatively impact on their functioning – for example, at school – it is less likely that they will meet criteria for a specific mental health diagnosis.

Could my own mental health issues be contributing to my child's behavior problems?

A child's temperament, mental health, and behavior are impacted by heredity and environmental factors. A positive family history of mental health diagnoses often increases a child's own risk of mental health diagnoses. In addition, if a parent is struggling to manage their own personal challenges, this can have an impact on the child. However, this does not mean that a parent with emotional challenges/mental health diagnoses cannot be an effective and positive parent. Recognizing and acknowledging your own personal challenges and seeking out appropriate treatment will often benefit your child.

My child's favorite activity is watching videos and playing with their electronic devices – will that "damage" him/her?

Electronic entertainment has increased in frequency for children, and monitoring what a child is watching/playing as well as the amount of time a child is spending engaged in electronics is an important part of parenting for the current generation of parents. This became even more challenging as a result of the COVID-19 pandemic, during which time virtual/online learning became a standard teaching method. Children may also be able to access inappropriate videos and games online, and parents of all children should be vigilant about monitoring the type of electronic entertainment in which their children are engaged. Even when the material being viewed is age appropriate, limiting the amount of time spent using electronics and encouraging outdoor activities, hands-on activities, and creative and social play-related activities is strongly recommended.

My relatives/friends have felt that my child is on the autism spectrum. They advised me to "fight" for this diagnosis. Is this good advice?

Some parents may feel more comfortable with the diagnosis of autism spectrum disorder than other developmental diagnoses, as awareness of this diagnosis has increased a great deal. Although part of a caregiver's job is to advocate for their child, they should be open to listening to the feedback from all the individuals involved in the child's life, including their primary care physician and teachers. As discussed in Chapter 4, a specific diagnosis such as ASD may allow a child access to specific services. However, there can be potential negative consequences of providing a child with a developmental diagnosis incorrectly. Seeking supports, resources, and services that may be available to children who are not felt to meet criteria for a specific diagnosis can often be beneficial. For example, a child who is shy, somewhat socially awkward, and may have some learning challenges may benefit from social skills assistance, even though they may not require more intensive interventions designed for children with ASD.

When does loving and caring about my child become suggestive of an "overprotective parent"?

It is natural and appropriate to love your children "more than life itself," but children need the experience of "falling down and getting up"; they need to learn to work with all types of people; and they need to make mistakes in order to develop problem-solving skills and work toward gradually increasing their independence.

Can you help me potty train my child?

The following are some tips for potty training.

- All children should be praised for any interest they show in using the potty/toilet.
- A child's developmental level should be used to gage when potty/toileting should be expected.
- Try your best not to make potty training a "battle."
- Reading children's potty books together in a playful interactive way can be beneficial.
- If a child is willing to urinate in the potty/toilet, but is resistant to moving their bowels, still praise your child for sitting on the toilet, using a pull-up/diaper in the bathroom area, assisting in flushing the toilet, etc.

My child's behavior is very difficult to manage and has caused a great deal of stress in our family. What should we do?

Families often benefit from working with a counselor to address a child's challenging behaviors. Learning the skills to manage behavioral problems and also exploring ways to improve family functioning can be addressed with a mental health professional.

Why does my child ask the same thing over and over? What can I do to stop this?

Children can perseverate ("get stuck") on things – this is sometimes a characteristic of a specific diagnosis (for example, autism, obsessive-compulsive disorder [OCD], anxiety, attention-deficit/hyperactivity disorder [ADHD]), and also characteristic of many typical children. You could try limit setting, which involves explaining to the child that they are only allowed to ask the same question or make the same statement a certain number of time. Respond to the question or statement each time, but remind the child how many more times they are allowed to ask the question; also remind the child that after they have reached the maximum number of times, a response will not be provided. Although there are several ways to handle a child's repetitive questions and requests, consistency in your responses is important.

Is it dangerous to medicate my young child?

Some medications are considered unsafe for children, and most pharmacologic information available about medications includes the age range for which the medication has been studied and is typically prescribed. Your child's physician will also be able to provide this information. The saying "start low and go slow" has been used to discuss the caution that should be taken when a trial of medication for a behavioral or psychiatric diagnosis is initiated for a child. Parents should also understand that a child's behavior naturally changes as they mature, whether or not they are treated with medication. Therefore, behavioral interventions and supports are typically the first line of treatment for children who demonstrate behavioral problems such as impulsivity and overactivity, and cautious trials of treatment with medication should be considered only if the child is experiencing great difficulty functioning in age-appropriate settings despite appropriate supports.

Can a special diet cure a developmental diagnosis such as ASD or ADHD?

Eating a well-balanced, healthy diet is important for everyone, and malnutrition and vitamin deficiencies are known to be associated with medical and developmental problems. Moreover, when a developmental disability is a result of an inborn error of metabolism or the inability to metabolize or absorb a specific nutrient (for example, phenylketonuria, maple syrup urine disease, glycogen storage disease, Celiac disease, etc.), a specific diet is necessary. There are clinicians and families who advocate specific diets for children with developmental disabilities that are not a result of an inborn error of metabolism or other gastrointestinal and endocrine diagnosis. However, there has been no definitive scientific evidence that a restrictive diet will "cure" developmental disabilities such as ASD, IDs, or ADHD in children who do not have a medical diagnosis for which a restrictive diet is necessary.

I think my child needs an individualized education program (IEP), but the school says she does not qualify. What should I do?

If the results of the testing completed by the school do not qualify your child for an IEP, you can consult with a professional to discuss the specific testing that was completed, the results of this testing, and whether additional testing would be appropriate. You can explore testing with an outside psychologist, neuropsychologist, or center-based multi-disciplinary team if it is felt that additional testing is indicated.

I feel like I am constantly battling with the school. Could it be that my child has a problem that I am not seeing? Are my expectations too high?

As a parent you want the best for your child. There are times when a school system may not be providing optimal education for a child. However, you should also sometimes take a step back and try to make a situation more positive by working with the school team to explore your concerns. Try to avoid the tendency to blame others for a perceived problem. Children need to learn from their parents' example that families and educators should attempt to work as a team to provide each child with an appropriate educational program.

What can I do to help my child thrive and maximize their potential?

It is our hope that this book has helped you answer this question. The book was inspired by the many children and families we have had the privilege to work with throughout our careers. Their stories, challenges, and triumphs expanded our understanding of child development and behavior and served as the heart of this work. By sharing our expertise, evidence-based information, and children's stories, we hope to offer practical, experience-based guidance to clinicians who are supporting children and families in their own careers. Whether a child's presentation falls within the broad range of typical development or points to a specific diagnosis, we firmly believe that every child has something valuable to teach those who are fortunate enough to be part of their journey.

Index

For Product Safety Concerns and Information please contact our EU
representative GPSR@taylorandfrancis.com
Taylor & Francis Verlag GmbH, Kaufingerstraße 24, 80331 München, Germany